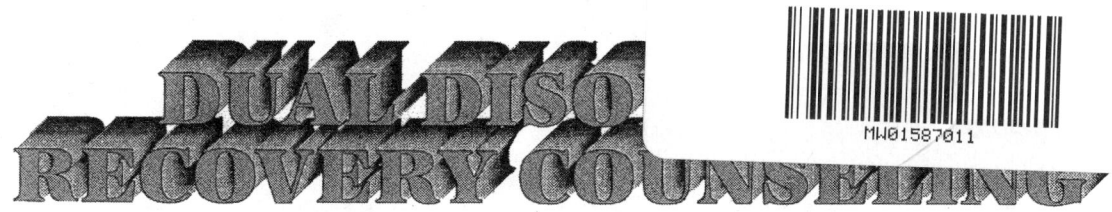

DUAL DISORDERS RECOVERY COUNSELING

by Dennis C. Daley, Ph.D.
and Michael E. Thase, M.D.

Third Edition

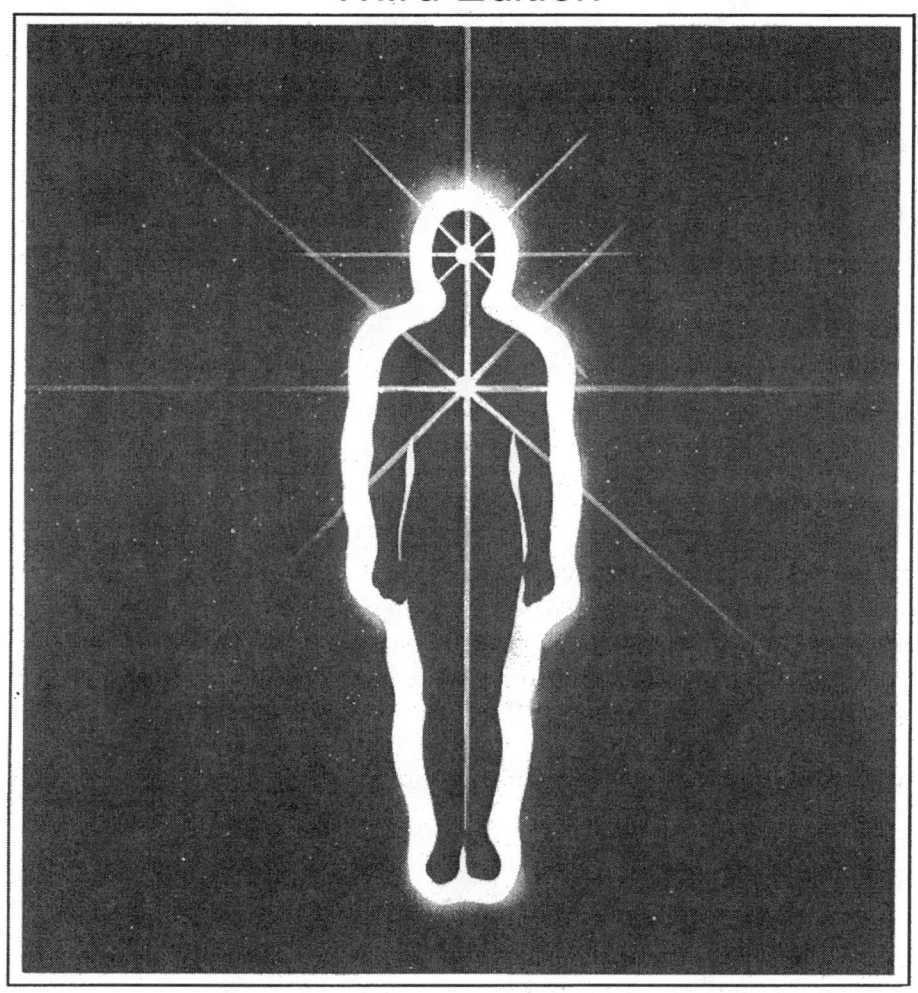

Integrated Treatment for Substance Use
and Mental Health Disorders

Foreword by Terence T. Gorski

Copyright © 1994, 2000, 2004 by Dennis C. Daley, Ph.D.

All rights reserved. No part of this book may be reproduced or transmitted in any form or by any means, including photocopying, without permission in writing from the author. While every precaution has been taken in the preparation of this book, the author and publisher assume no responsibility for errors or omissions. Neither is any liability assumed for damages resulting from the use of the information in this guide.

Additional copies of this book are available from the publisher:

Herald House/Independence Press
1001 W. Walnut
P.O. Box 390
Independence, MO 64051-0390
Phone: 1-800-767-8181 or (816) 521-3015
Fax: (816) 521-3066
Web site: *www.relapse.org*

Other clinician manuals, books, guides, and workbooks on substance use disorders, mental illness, or dual disorders authored by Dennis C. Daley, Ph.D., are available at *www.drdenniscdaley.com*.

Printed in the United States of America
ISBN 9780830911493

"Drs. Daley and Thase present an integrated model of treatment for co-occurring disorders that synthesizes the empirical literature and their extensive clinical experiences. We have been using their integrated model of care at Western Psychiatric Institute and Clinic for nearly two decades. Their treatment model is used in many treatment programs throughout the United States and other countries. I highly recommend this informative and practical book to clinicians working with clients who have both substance use and psychiatric disorders."
—David J. Kupfer, M.D., Thomas Detre Professor and Chair, Department of Psychiatry, University of Pittsburgh Medical Center; Pittsburgh, Pennsylvania

"Dennis Daley, in collaboration with Michael Thase, has developed a manual for addiction counselors (and other practitioners) on dual diagnosis recovery counseling that is a 'must read' for every clinician engaged in doing this work. Dr. Daley is well known for developing premier materials to help counselors develop comfort and competency in working with clients with co-occurring mental health disorders. The current manual builds on this past work and creates what I would consider to be the definitive textbook for addiction professionals seeking to understand their scope of practice in individual and group counseling in any program setting and to have access to a comprehensive range of adaptable materials that cover every aspect of dual diagnosis recovery counseling. As we become increasingly aware that 'dual diagnosis is an expectation' in every treatment setting, Dr. Daley's manual will become an 'expectation' in the library of every addiction program."
—Ken Minkoff, M.D., Medical Director, Arbour-Choate Health Management, Clinical Assistant Professor of Psychiatry, Harvard Medical School

"I strongly recommend this outstanding counseling manual, *Dual Disorders Recovery Counseling* (Third Edition) by Dr. Dennis Daley and Dr. Michael Thase. The material presented in this comprehensive manual provides an evidence-based and comprehensive integration of treatment for patients with co-occurring substance abuse and mental health problems (dual disorders). It is an excellent resource for clinicians and counselors who work on the front line with dual diagnosis patients."
—G. Alan Marlatt, Ph.D., Professor and Director, Addictive Behaviors Research Center, University of Washington

"The importance of knowledgeable, highly skilled clinicians to provide integrated treatment for individuals with co-occurring psychiatric and addictive disorders cannot be overstated. However, in practice, the need for qualified clinicians far exceeds their availability. The third edition of *Dual Disorders Recovery Counseling: Integrated Treatment for Substance Use and Mental Health Disorders* is a valuable manual for any clinician who works with, or is interested in working with, people with co-occurring disorders. In this manual, Drs. Daley and Thase provide essential information for any clinician who wants to lay a strong foundation on which to build higher levels of therapeutic skill and competence."
—Patricia L. Valentine, Deputy Director for Behavioral Health, Allegheny County Department of Human Services

"This book for clinicians by Drs. Daley and Thase is based on sound clinical studies. Their integrated treatment approach produces outcomes that are far above the norm for clients with substance use and psychiatric disorders. Their work is at the highest level and yet is easy to use for frontline clinicians. We have been using this treatment manual and Dr. Daley's recovery manuals for clients and families throughout our treatment continuum with excellent results. This book is one of the most effective tools for treatment of co-occurring disorders."

—Natalie Honeycutt, M.Ed., LPC, MHSP, EAP Coordinator,
Frontier Health; Grey, Tennessee

"This practical treatment manual provides a framework for treating clients with addiction and psychiatric disorders. It reviews individual, group, and family applications of an integrated treatment model. The group component is quite extensive. I have been using Dr. Daley's clinical and client recovery materials for many years in our programs at McLean Hospital. I highly recommend this book by Drs. Daley and Thase."

—Bill Lopez, MPH, Partial Hospital Program Coordinator,
McLean Hospital of Harvard Medical School

"We have treated thousands of clients in our programs using this model of integrated treatment. Clients find this approach informative, hopeful, and helpful in learning about recovery and developing skills to manage their dual disorders. The group component of this model is easy to adapt to various clinical populations."

—Marybeth Grundler, BA, CAC, Partial Hospital Therapist,
Center for Psychiatric and Chemical Dependency Services

Contents

Foreword by Terence T. Gorski 7
Preface 10
Acknowledgment 12
Chapter 1: Overview of Dual Disorders and Treatment 13
Chapter 2: Recovery from Dual Disorders 19
Chapter 3: Format of DDRC 33
Chapter 4: Counselor Training and Supervision 36
Chapter 5: The Assessment Process 46
Chapter 6: Motivation and Treatment Adherence 50
Chapter 7: Individual Treatment 54
Chapter 8: Role of the Family and Significant Others in Treatment ... 67
Chapter 9: Overview of Group Treatments 71
Chapter 10: Dual Recovery Psychoeducational Group Topics 81
    1. Overview of Dual Disorders 84
    2. Understanding Psychiatric Illness 87
    3. Understanding Addiction 89
    4. Effects of Dual Disorders 92
    5. Medical Effects of Alcohol and Drugs 94
    6. Withdrawal from Alcohol and Other Drugs 96
    7. Alcohol and Other Depressants 98
    8. Cocaine and Other Stimulants 100
    9. Heroin and Other Opiates 102
    10. Psychosocial Effects of Substance Disorders 104
    11. How to Use Treatment: Keys to Successful Recovery 106
    12. Phases of Recovery 108
    13. Developing a Problem List 111
    14. Setting Treatment Goals 113
    15. Advantages of Recovery 115
    16. Denial in Addiction and Psychiatric Illness 117

17. Roadblocks in Recovery 119
18. Recovery from Dual Disorders 121
19. Managing Cravings for Alcohol or Drugs 123
20. Managing People, Places, Events, and Things 125
21. Managing Persistent Psychiatric Symptoms 127
22. Managing Anger 129
23. Managing Anxiety and Worry 131
24. Managing Boredom 134
25. Managing Depression 136
26. Managing Guilt and Shame 139
27. Sharing Positive Feelings in Recovery 141
28. Dual Disorders and the Family 143
29. Impact of Disorders on Children 146
30. Impact of Dual Disorders on Relationships 148
31. Saying No to Getting High 150
32. Resisting Pressures to Stop Taking Psychiatric Medications 152
33. Building a Recovery Network 154
34. Self-Help Programs 156
35. Changing Negative or Inaccurate Thinking 158
36. Changing Self-Defeating Behaviors 160
37. Changing Personality Problems 163
38. Developing Spirituality 165
39. Using a Daily Plan in Recovery 167
40. Financial Issues in Dual Recovery 169
41. Managing Relapse Warning Signs 171
42. Managing High-Risk Relapse Factors 173
43. Coping with Emergencies and Setbacks 175

Endnotes 177
Reference List 182
Videos for Client and Family Education 198
World Wide Web-Based Resources 200

Foreword

Many people suffer from the dual disorders of a psychiatric illness and a substance use disorder (chemical dependency). These dual disorders are serious because they can lead to relapse if they are not properly treated.

For many years I have believed that there needs to be a comprehensive guide for dealing with dual disorders. When I became familiar with Dr. Dennis Daley's work, I was impressed. I had the privilege of presenting with him at an NIDA panel of experts and asked him if he would be interested in publishing an expanded version of his model complete with session-by-session breakdowns of his group protocol. I was delighted when he agreed because his work is concrete, specific, and field-tested over a number of years with dual disorder patients. Dr. Daley not only has considerable experience in providing clinical care and developing programs, he has been involved in over ten funded research projects as an investigator, trainer, and consultant. All of these projects have been in the area of addiction medicine or dual disorders treatment. He also has more than two hundred and thirty-five publications including journal articles, books and chapters, educational videos, and recovery guides and workbooks for clients, families, and children.

I was also delighted that he invited Michael Thase, M.D., to coauthor this manual. Dr. Thase is a highly regarded researcher and clinician in the treatment of mood disorders. He has considerable expertise in both pharmacotherapy and cognitive therapy. Dr. Thase has extensive research experience in the areas of mood disorders, addiction, and mood disorders combined with addiction. He has published more than three hundred papers in scientific journals or book chapters. Drs. Daley and Thase and their colleagues have developed numerous specialty dual disorders treatment programs at the University of Pittsburgh Medical Center at Western Psychiatric Institute and Clinic (WPIC) in Pittsburgh, Pennsylvania.

I would like to use this foreword as an opportunity to summarize the basic principles that can improve the effectiveness of treatment of dual diagnosis clients. Because they are so compatible with the operationalized procedures of Drs. Daley and Thase, these principles will act as an excellent introduction to their work.

Treatment Planning for Dual Disorders

Effective treatment planning for dual diagnosis clients includes the following components: (1) integrated treatment for managing the symptoms of chemical dependency and psychiatric disorders, (2) physical interventions for managing medical problems, (3) cognitive strategies for changing irrational thoughts, (4) affective strategies for changing unmanageable feelings, (5) behavioral strategies for changing self-defeating behaviors, and (6) social/situational strategies for changing lifestyle.

Coexisting Disorders

Dual disorders are best conceptualized as coexisting disorders that are interrelated and require integrated treatment. It is generally not helpful to try to determine which disorder is primary and which is secondary. It is more productive to profile the client's physical, psychological, and social symptoms and then develop a treatment plan to stabilize the symptoms of all disorders.

As a general rule, clients must stop using alcohol and drugs of abuse for treatment to be most effective. Chemical dependency is present in 40 to 60 percent of all mental health clients. All mental health clients must be evaluated for a substance use disorder (SUD).

Clients with psychiatric disorders cannot recover from their SUD until they achieve a stable mental status. This requires the stabilization of the symptoms that interfere with rational thought, emotional management, and behavior self-control. In some cases the stabilization of the mental disorder may require the uses of psychoactive medication.

Effective clinical systems integrate a biopsychosocial model of diagnosis, a developmental model of recovery for treatment planning, and relapse prevention strategies for identifying and managing the problems that lead to relapse.

The Biopsychosocial Model

The biopsychosocial model for dual disorders targets physical, psychological, and social symptoms related to client's disorders. The physical symptoms often involve brain chemistry imbalances that can be corrected with the use of psychotropic medication. The psychological symptoms include problems with thinking, emotional management, and behavior. The social symptoms include problems with work, friends, and family.

The Developmental Model of Recovery divides recovery into six stages: transition, stabilization, early recovery, middle recovery, late recovery, and maintenance. Each phase has specific tasks for the client and interventions for the clinician.

Relapse Prevention Therapy (RPT)

Relapse is a possibility for clients at any stage of recovery. Any stressor or sudden change can elevate stress and trigger relapse. RPT is a specialized method that helps clients identify and manage relapse warning signs and intervene early should relapse occur. For most dual recovery clients, there is a process called reciprocal relapse. Relapse into chemical addiction will usually trigger a relapse into the mental disorders. Relapse into the symptoms of the mental disorder will usually activate craving for alcohol and other drugs.

Dennis Daley's Dual Diagnosis Workbook for Clients

As you will see, *Dual Disorders Recovery Counseling* and the companion guide for clients, *Dual Diagnosis Workbook*, are powerful resources for bringing these concepts to life. The counseling manual and client workbook have been carefully developed and revised based on the empirical literature and the clinical experiences of Drs. Daley and Thase. The methods have been shown to work. I am impressed with these books because they are practical tools that can be used with clients and their families. The clinical principles are sound, and they are presented in a clear, concise, and easy-to-understand way. If used as designed they can form the basis of effective dual diagnosis treatment. I wish you well in exploring the concepts and procedures and putting them to work in helping clients and their families recover.

—Terence T. Gorski

Preface

In behavioral health care there is increased focus on treating clients who suffer from the dual disorders (also called co-occurring disorders) of a psychiatric illness and a substance use disorder (SUD). While traditional methods of treatment for psychiatric or SUDs have helped, many clients have not experienced the full benefits because the focus was primarily on either the psychiatric illness or the SUD.

This manual was written to provide a framework for clinicians who take care of dual diagnosis clients. It is intended to be a practical manual that can be adapted to current counseling practices in various treatment settings. While we provide information on topics, issues, and problems to discuss in individual sessions or treatment groups, this manual is not meant to serve as a "cookbook" approach that is to be used in a rigid fashion. We believe that while treatment manuals are valuable for clinicians, the use of them does not ensure competence and effectiveness. Manuals are simply "tools" that help clinicians in their work with clients. The "art" of treatment requires the clinician to develop rapport and a therapeutic alliance with the client, work together to identify problems and treatment goals, and collaborate in resolving problems or impasses in the treatment relationship. Many therapists and counselors are savvy and creative when it comes to adapting treatment manuals to meet their clients' needs.

The impetus for this treatment manual came from numerous experiences. First, along with several colleagues from around the country, Dr. Daley was invited by the National Institute of Drug Abuse (NIDA) to a one-day meeting where each participant presented a "Counseling Approach" relevant to the problems of addiction. This meeting was moderated by Lisa Onken, Ph.D., and Jack Blaine, M.D., from NIDA, and Kathleen Carroll, Ph.D., from Yale University. The intent was to have presenters "concretize" treatment approaches. This revised *Dual Disorders Recovery Counseling* manual is a significant expansion of the version presented at this meeting using the format suggested by NIDA for writing clinical manuals.

Second, we were involved in a National Institute of Drug Abuse multisite clinical trial "Psychosocial Treatments of Cocaine Addiction." Three individual manuals and one group treatment manual were used. Dr. Daley cowrote the group manual for this study and contributed to one of the individual treatment manuals. He has also written treatment manuals for other funded studies. Dr. Thase has written cognitive behavioral treatment manuals for inpatients and outpatients with mood disorders, including those with co-occurring substance use disorders. The use of evidenced-based treatment manuals has been found useful by clinicians from a variety of professional disciplines.

Third, at Western Psychiatric Institute and Clinic (WPIC) of the University of Pittsburgh School of Medicine, we have been involved in developing and implementing dual diagnosis treatment programs in inpatient, partial hospital, and outpatient settings for almost two decades. WPIC was one of the first institutions in the United States to develop specialized treatment programs for dual diagnosis clients in both psychiatric and addiction treatment settings. We have changed our programs based on the empirical and clinical literature and our experience treating thousands of clients with all types and combinations of disorders.

Fourth, our clinical work and research has included providing supervision to professionals from a variety of disciplines. We have gained an understanding of the knowledge and skill needs of clinicians who work with dual diagnosis clients. We also developed adherence scales for use in supervision, which are adaptable to clients not involved in clinical trials (see Chapter 4).

Fifth, for several years Dr. Daley regularly met with clients in several dual disorders treatment programs to elicit their feedback on what they liked best and least about these programs. This input has enabled us to learn what clients find helpful in their recovery.

Sixth, we have written workbooks and recovery manuals for clients and families, including a comprehensive manual by Dr. Daley titled *Dual Diagnosis Workbook: Recovery Strategies for Substance Use and Mental Health Disorders*. This counseling manual describes ways this client workbook can be used. Most of the sections in the workbook are described in Chapter 10 of this manual. Written evaluations by clients and focus groups indicate that workbooks and recovery materials are found by clients as being very informative and helpful in their recovery.

Seventh, in our teaching and lecturing at the University of Pittsburgh Medical Center and throughout the United States, Canada, and Europe, we talk with many professionals in mental health, substance abuse, and dual diagnosis treatment settings. We have heard the problems, concerns, and needs of professionals who treat clients with dual disorders, and are well aware of the current challenges faced in treating dual disorder clients.

This manual can also serve as a resource guide for clinicians. The bibliography is extensive and includes books, treatment manuals, book chapters, and journal articles on psychiatric, substance use, and dual disorders. Suggestions are provided in the group curriculum in Chapter 10 for written materials and videos to use with clients. A list of Web-based resources is provided at the end of this manual where additional materials can be found on all topics discussed in this manual.

There are several limitations of this manual. First, it does not review specific criteria for psychiatric or SUDs. We assume the reader is either familiar with these disorders or has access to the American Psychiatric Association's *Diagnostic and Statistical Manual of Mental Disorders (DSM IV TR)*, which reviews specific diagnostic criteria. Second, although this current manual was written to provide a practical overview of a model of counseling, it does not address gender or cultural diversity issues. The reader is encouraged to continuously consider gender and ethnicity issues in clinical practice. Finally, while this book provides a framework for conducting DDRC sessions it does not address the clinical nuances and issues specific to the many different types of psychiatric disorders. We assume that counselors using this manual will have access to training and/or supervision that will assist them in understanding how to adapt interventions discussed to different clinical populations and treatment settings diagnostic groups of client. Despite these or other limitations, we believe that this practical manual will aid clinicians in helping clients with dual disorders.

Dennis C. Daley, Ph.D.
Michael E. Thase, M.D.

Acknowledgment

We wish to thank Cindy Hurney, administrative manager for Addiction Medicine Services at Western Psychiatric Institute and Clinic of the University of Pittsburgh Medical Center, for all her help in designing and updating this treatment manual.

Chapter 1
Overview of Dual Disorders and Treatment

Introduction and Overview

There is significant research showing that many clients suffer from the dual disorders of psychiatric illness and a substance use disorder (SUD, also referred to as chemical dependency or addiction).[1] Many books focus on treatment approaches for dual disorders.[2] For maximum benefit, treatment should address both disorders in an integrated way.

Dual Disorders Recovery Counseling (DDRC) was developed to provide a framework for integrated treatment. DDRC is flexible, comprehensive, and adaptable to clients in a variety of psychiatric or addiction treatment settings. Our model draws on information from the addiction,[3] psychiatric[4] and dual diagnosis[5] literature including individual, group and family approaches, skills training, psychoeducation, relapse prevention, psychiatric rehabilitation, addiction rehabilitation, and mutual support groups.

Psychiatric disorders vary in their severity and effects on the client and family. While some disorders are chronic and persistent with multiple adverse sequelae, other disorders are experienced as a single episode and do not have implications for long-term involvement in recovery. SUDs also vary in terms of severity, chronicity, and adverse effects on the client and family and treatment implications.

The problems and recovery needs of a particular client will depend on the type and severity of the substance use and psychiatric disorders, ego strength and psychological functioning, social and family support systems, and internal motivation to change. Although everyone can change in some ways, the more chronically impaired clients have more difficulty achieving or maintaining sobriety, managing psychiatric symptoms, and coping with life problems caused or worsened by their disorders.

Dual Disorders Paradigms

There are three paradigms for understanding and treating dual disorders: parallel, sequential, and integrated.[6] The parallel model involves the client receiving treatment for the psychiatric disorder in a mental health program and treatment for the SUD in an addiction medicine program. Involvement in separate agencies increases the odds of poor adherence, as the client has to adjust to two treatment philosophies, develop relationships with several professionals, and attend services at different locations. It is not unusual, for example, for treatment philosophies and expectations to vary between mental health and addiction medicine treatment agencies.

The sequential model involves addressing and stabilizing the most acute disorder first, then addressing the other disorder. Since symptoms often overlap (it is not easy to distinguish between primary and secondary disorders), this approach may put the client in a situation where specific symptoms are not sufficiently addressed. For example, a dual diagnosis client with depression receiving services from an addiction medicine program could be in a situation where depression is seen as secondary and not addressed, thus causing undue suffering for the client.

The integrated model is viewed as the most effective of the three models. While all three approaches may be helpful for a specific client, evidence suggests that clients receiving integrated treatment have higher rates of treatment adherence and improved clinical outcomes compared to those receiving parallel or sequential treatment, particularly clients with more persistent and chronic forms of mental illness.[7]

Goals and Objectives of DDRC

The goals of the DDRC model are as follows:

1. Achievement and maintenance of abstinence from alcohol or other drugs of abuse. Alternatively, for clients unable or unwilling to work toward total abstinence, reduction of amount and frequency of use and concomitant biopsychosocial sequelae associated with substance use.
2. Stabilization from acute psychiatric symptoms.
3. Resolution or reduction of psychiatric symptoms and problems and learning to manage persistent symptoms of psychiatric illness.
4. Improved cognitive, behavioral, and interpersonal coping skills.
5. Improvement in functioning: physical, emotional, social, family, interpersonal, occupational, academic, spiritual, financial, and legal.
6. Positive lifestyle change and improvement in the quality of life.
7. Early intervention in the process of relapse to either substance use or psychiatric disorder.

Rationale and Mechanism of Action for DDRC Model

This treatment model is based on the rationale that integrated treatment is the best approach to helping the client with dual disorders. Although the client may use a specific form of treatment at times (i.e., an addiction rehabilitation program to initiate abstinence and set the foundation of recovery), integrated treatment focuses on both psychiatric and substance use issues. This dual focus reduces the chances that an untreated disorder will increase vulnerability to relapse to another disorder.

The DDRC approach involves the following interventions:

1. Motivating the client to seek detoxification or inpatient treatment if symptoms warrant and facilitating an involuntary commitment for psychiatric care if needed.
2. Educating the client and family about psychiatric illness, addictive illness, treatment, and the recovery process.
3. Helping the client increase self-awareness so information regarding dual disorders can be understood in a personal way.

4. Supporting the client's efforts at recovery and providing a sense of hope regarding positive change.
5. Helping the client identify problems and areas of change.
6. Helping the client develop or improve the ability to problem solve and develop recovery coping skills.
7. Facilitating a medication evaluation and compliance. This requires close collaboration with a psychiatrist.
8. Engaging the family in the treatment process when appropriate.
9. Referring the client for other services (case management, medical, social, vocational, economic, housing).

Agents of Change

The DDRC model assumes that change occurs as a result of the client's relationship with the clinician and treatment team. A therapeutic alliance is critical to help the client remain active in treatment and engaged in the recovery process. Community support systems, treatment groups, and self-help programs also serve as agents of change for clients. For the more chronically and persistently mentally ill clients, a case manager is an important agent in the change process.

Although the client works on intrapersonal and interpersonal issues in recovery, medications facilitate this process by attenuating acute symptoms, improving mood, cognitive abilities, or impulse control. For example, a severely depressed client may be unable to focus on using cognitive or behavioral interventions until she experiences relief from her depressed symptoms; a psychotic client will not be able to focus on abstinence from drugs until his psychotic symptoms are under control.

Etiology and Causative Factors

Both psychiatric and addictive illnesses are biopsychosocial disorders. These are caused or maintained by a variety of biological, psychological, and social factors.[8]

Biological factors include genetic influences, differences in the structure of the brain or in the neurotransmitters in the brain. Many psychiatric disorders such as bipolar illness and schizophrenia, and substance use disorders run in families. These disorders are more prevalent among offspring who have a parent or sibling with one of these disorders. The brain structure or the ways the neurotransmitters work differs in individuals with certain types of disorders compared to others who do not have these disorders. Many substances mimic neurotransmitters. Over time, alcohol or drugs can "hijack" the limbic system ("reward pathway"). The "feeling" caused by repeatedly using these substances can surpass that experienced by natural methods of gaining pleasure (e.g., from sports, accomplishments, experiences). The result is that the person craves substances and continues to use despite the adverse consequences such use may cause.

Psychological factors include belief systems, personality traits, conditioned responses, and the ability to cope with life problems and stresses. Some individuals are more vulnerable to ordinary life stresses than others are. Others are much more resilient and able to bounce back from life problems and stresses.

Social factors contributing to these disorders include environmental influences (family and community), and personal experiences. For example, a significant loss of a relationship can contribute to depression or the need to escape emotional pain through the use of substances. Acceptance of drug use within a culture may contribute to increased availability of substance use.

Relationships between Psychiatric and Substance Use Disorders

There are several possible relationships between psychiatric illness and substance use disorders.[9] These include the following:

1. Axis I and II psychopathology serve as a risk factor for addictive disorders. The odds of having an addictive disorder among individuals with a mental illness are 2.7 according to the National Institute of Mental Health's Epidemiologic Catchment Area (ECA) survey. Compared to a person without a mental disorder, an individual with a mental health disorder is almost three times more likely to have a substance use disorder.

2. Addiction is a risk factor for psychiatric illness. The odds of having a psychiatric disorder among those with a drug use disorder are 4.5 according to the ECA survey. This means that drug abusers are four and one-half times more likely to have a psychiatric diagnosis compared to non-drug abusers.

3. Clients with psychiatric disorders are more vulnerable than others to the adverse effects of alcohol or other drugs. For example, the use of marijuana or hallucinogens can be much more harmful to a person with schizophrenia or borderline personality disorder than a person who does not have these disorders.

4. The use of drugs can precipitate an underlying psychiatric condition. For example, PCP or cocaine use may trigger a first manic episode in a vulnerable individual.

5. Psychopathology may modify the course of an addictive disorder in terms of:

    - Rapidity of course: "male-limited" alcoholics with antisocial behaviors have earlier onset of addiction compared to "milieu-limited" alcoholics.[10]

    - Response to treatment: dual diagnosis clients often drop out of treatment early, and many fail to continue care once discharged from an inpatient hospital or residential treatment program.[11]

    - Symptom picture and long-term outcome: "high psychiatric severity" clients do worse than "low psychiatric severity" clients;[12] there is a strong association between relapse and psychiatric impairment among opiate addicts and some association between relapse and psychiatric impairment among alcoholics.[13]

6. Psychiatric symptoms can develop in the course of chronic intoxications. For example, psychosis may follow PCP use or chronic stimulant use; or suicidality and depression may follow a cocaine crash.

7. Psychiatric symptoms can emerge as a consequence of chronic use of substances or a relapse. For example, depression may be caused by an awareness of the losses associated with addiction or after a relapse.

8. Substance-using behavior and psychiatric symptoms, regardless of which came first, will become linked over the course of time.

9. The addictive disorder and psychiatric disorder can develop at different points in time. For example, a bipolar client may become hooked on drugs years after being stable from a manic disorder; or an alcoholic may develop panic disorder or major depression long after being sober.

10. Symptoms of one disorder can contribute to relapse of the other disorder and the need for hospitalization.[14] For example, an increase in anxiety or hallucinations may lead a client with schizophrenia to alcohol or other drug use to ameliorate symptoms; a cocaine or alcohol binge may lead to depressive symptoms or suicidality.

Challenges for Clinicians and Providers

We see the following as the challenges facing clinicians and treatment systems providing care to clients with dual disorders.

1. *Convey helpful attitudes.* We have consulted with numerous professionals about their frustration and negative attitudes in dealing with psychiatrically ill clients who have substance use disorders. Anger, frustration, and judgmentalism are commonly expressed. Such negative reactions and feelings must be contained. To be effective, clinicians must understand and accept these clients as being ill and convey genuine concern and empathy.

2. *Understand illness from the "inside out."* Try to understand what it is like to be dependent on substances, or want to use alcohol or drugs so bad that you are willing to risk losing your family, job, or health. Think about what it feels like to have a psychiatric disorder and how this affects your self-image, ability to function, or vision of the future.

3. *Develop client and family centered standards of care.* A panel of national experts on dual disorders developed standards of care, practice guidelines, workforce competencies, and training curricula.[15] This panel recommended that clinical care for clients and families should be:

    - *Welcoming:* services should be consumer centered; caregivers need to show empathy toward clients and optimism about their chances for recovery, even those who struggle with motivation to change and make minimal changes.

    - *Accessible:* clients with any combination of disorders need to be accommodated in treatment systems, regardless of their level of readiness to change.

- *Integrated:* clinicians should be competent in both mental health and substance abuse treatment approaches so that integrated care is provided.
- *Continuous:* when possible, the treatment team should maintain continuous contact with the client throughout all episodes.
- *Comprehensive:* treatment services should be sensitive to cultural and gender issues, and offer a range of clinical and ancillary services to address the needs and problems of the client.

4. *Think family, not just consumer.* Families and children are adversely affected by dual disorders. Helping the client examine the impact of disorders on the family, eliciting support from the family, and providing education, support, and therapy to the family are some of the ways in which families can be helped.

5. *Provide integrated assessment and treatment services.* A comprehensive assessment takes time and effort and is used to guide treatment planning. An assessment must include a substance use, psychiatric, psychosocial, and medical history. Integrated treatment services focus on both substance use and psychiatric issues, acknowledging that each affects the other.

6. *Integrate evidenced-based treatments into clinical care.* Many scientific studies have been conducted to determine the efficacy of various treatments for psychiatric illness, addiction, or dual disorders.[16] Clinicians should be aware of evidenced-based treatments and integrate these in clinical care. A later section in this chapter provides a listing of empirically-based treatments. Our recommendation is that mental health professionals learn one model of addiction treatment and integrate appropriate interventions into their daily work. Likewise, addiction medicine professionals can learn one model of treatment for psychiatric illness and integrate this into their clinical care with dual diagnosis clients.

7. *Improve linkages between different levels of care.* Clients who fail to engage in the next level of care following completion of another level are at risk for relapse. For example, psychiatric inpatients who enter ambulatory care and adhere to an adequate dose of treatment are less likely to be rehospitalized than those who fail to continue care after hospital discharge. Many effective motivational and adherence improvement interventions exist, which can help clinicians improve these linkages.[17]

8. *Utilize strategies to improve adherence to treatment.* Clients benefit from treatment to the extent they remain in it for a sufficient period of time. No short-term treatments exist for dual disorders, particularly for clients who have more serious and persistent forms of mental illness. There are many systems and clinical-related strategies that improve adherence. Clinicians should become familiar with adherence-improving strategies and integrate these into their clinical work.[18]

Chapter 2
Recovery from Dual Disorders

Recovery

Recovery is the process of managing dual disorders over time. It involves making changes in physical, emotional, psychological, cognitive, interpersonal, family, social, or spiritual domains of functioning.[1] DDRC is one of the first manuals to advocate a "recovery-oriented" approach to the treatment of dual disorders. It is based on the assumption that clients need to assume control over their recovery in order to manage their disorders and make changes. Recovery is facilitated by the use of mutual support programs such as AA, NA, DRA, and other mental health programs.

Phases or Stages of Change

Researchers and clinicians have outlined phases or stages of the change process for psychological problems,[2] addictive disorders,[3] psychiatric disorders,[4] and dual disorders.[5] Although each model of the change process is somewhat different, each model views change as occurring in phases. Each phase involves recovery tasks for the client and interventions for professionals providing treatment.

The DDRC model is based on the assumption that there are six possible phases of treatment that clients may progress through over time. These phases are "rough guidelines" that delineate issues that clients deal with pertinent to their disorders at various points in recovery. Because of the variability of severity and chronicity of dual disorders, motivation to change, internal resources, and external support, not all clients will progress through these phases in the same manner or in a linear fashion. Some clients will move back and forth between phases as their conditions worsen or improve. Others will never move much beyond the first several phases. These phases provide a clinical and recovery framework from which to approach dual disorders treatment.

Following is a discussion of these phases and the approximate time a client may be in each phase. The time frame is very rough because there is variation among individuals. Case examples are provided at the end of each phase, illustrating how clients successfully negotiate a phase and how others have difficulty moving through a phase. As managed care continues to influence the duration of treatment, the time available to treat clients is likely to shorten. This will require clinicians to limit the number of sessions provided, which in turn influences the focus of therapeutic interventions.

Phase 1—Transition and Engagement

This phase involves becoming engaged in treatment, either voluntarily or as a result of an involuntary commitment. It involves recognition by the client of an inability to control the use of substances. It also involves recognition that the psychiatric disorder requires treatment. In cases of involuntarily commitment due to psychiatric decompensation, recognition may not occur until there is stability of the acute symptoms.

Alcohol or drug use can contribute to a new episode of psychiatric illness following a period of remission. Alternatively, substance use may worsen existing symptoms such as depression, mania, psychosis, suicidality, anxiety, panic, threatening behaviors toward others, or an inability to function and take care of basic needs. In some cases, alcohol or drug use may "mask" psychiatric symptoms, prolonging the client's engagement in treatment.

During this phase, the client recognizes that an untreated psychiatric disorder interferes with his motivation to recover and ability to remain sober. The client comes to grips with mixed feelings about recovery, accepting that the healthy part wants to stop using substances, and the sick or addicted part does not want to stop using. The same is true for the psychiatric illness—the client accepts that part of him needs help and part of him does not think help is needed.

The family should get involved in assessment and treatment early in the process. This is best accomplished by assuming that family involvement is important and expected, then conveying to the client that the treatment team would like to invite the family for sessions. The client can be told that the more the family understands about dual disorders and recovery, the more supportive they can be for the client. The counselor can stress that family members who attend sessions find it helpful in addressing their questions, concerns, and feelings. Family members can provide helpful information to professionals who care for the client, provide emotional support to the client, and they can gain much from treatment for themselves.

Engagement of the family requires patience and persistence. Outreach efforts are often needed to get the family to attend sessions. When families attend individual family sessions with one or more members of the treatment team, they can be asked specific questions about the client's functioning within the family. The family can be encouraged to share their questions, concerns, and feelings. Families can be invited to multiple family groups or family psychoeducational workshops to gain information about dual disorders, the recovery process, treatment approaches, and their role in treatment. These services give family members a chance to be heard and gain support from others.

The client begins to accept the need for a recovery program that involves a combination of professional treatment and self-help programs such as AA, NA, CA, DRA, or other mental health support groups. The client learns that help and support from others is needed to recover from dual disorders. The client's motivation to change initially may be "external" as he gets involved in recovery due to the problems caused by his disorders. Or the client may engage in treatment because he was forced or pressured to accept help by the family, an employer, the court system, a health care or social service professional, or a friend.

This phase may take up to several weeks or longer, although for some it takes much longer. Some clients enter treatment only to drop out early. If a client makes a commitment to stay in recovery, even if he feels his motivation is questionable, he puts himself in a position to benefit from it. Many people need time to develop their motivation to recover, and staying in treatment "buys time" for them to develop motivation and see the benefits of recovery.

> *Case #1: Michael is a 34-year-old married employed father of two children who was involuntarily committed to a psychiatric hospital following a manic episode. During this episode, Michael's judgment became severely impaired. He became irrational and threatened to kick his wife and children out of their home, insisted he was going to take over a business in another state and quit going to work. He started drinking after two years of sobriety and eventually was arrested for trying to solicit teenagers to have sex with him. The police initiated an involuntary commitment when it was clear that Michael was out of touch with reality and a threat to others. Once his mood and behavior stabilized during his hospitalization, Michael realized the seriousness of his condition and the impact on his behavior and agreed to continue outpatient treatment. He recognized that his bipolar illness contributed to an alcohol relapse and agreed he needed to abstain from alcohol. During inpatient treatment, his family attended several family psychoeducational groups to gain information about dual disorders, the impact on families, and recovery strategies. He also had sessions with his family and members of his treatment team to discuss the impact of his behaviors on his wife and kids, their feelings and reactions, and ongoing recovery strategies. His wife was encouraged to resume Al-Anon participation, as this had been helpful to her in the past.*

> *Case #2: Charles is a 41-year-old divorced father of three with a long history of multiple psychiatric hospitalizations, rehabilitation programs, and outpatient treatment. He has been treated for recurrent depression, antisocial personality disorders, heroin addiction, alcoholism, and more recently, crack/cocaine addiction. Although Charles has had a period of sobriety for more than one year and periods of stable psychiatric functioning in the past, since getting addicted to crack two years ago he's been unable to stay drug free for more than a month. During the past two years, he's been hospitalized three times for depression and suicide attempts. Unfortunately, Charles always drops out of outpatient or partial hospital programs before becoming engaged in treatment. His pattern is to attend a few outpatient or partial hospital sessions with many cancellations and no-shows. He usually returns briefly to treatment when he "needs" something or is in a crisis resulting from his drug uses or depressive symptomatology. Even multiple efforts at outreach have had a limited impact on Charles's ability to engage in treatment.*

Phase 2—Stabilization from Acute Symptoms of Dual Disorders

This phase involves stabilizing from the acute psychiatric symptoms and may last weeks to months. The client may receive medications to stabilize acute psychiatric symptoms. It may take several weeks or longer for medications to reduce or eliminate symptoms. This requires patience and a willingness to stick with treatment even when the client feels frustrated because symptoms are not improving quickly enough. In some cases, stabilizing from an episode of illness is a relatively smooth process. In other cases, it is more complex and takes longer. The counselor also needs to be patient and provide support and education to help the client through this process.

The stabilization phase involves getting alcohol and drugs out of the client's system and adjusting to being substance free. For some people, detoxification is needed to break the cycle of addictive substance use. Acute symptoms of withdrawal usually last a few days to a week. The specific withdrawal symptoms experienced depend on the amount and types of substances used and length of use. Protracted or post-acute withdrawal symptoms may last for weeks or longer. If the client's body was accustomed to heavy use of alcohol or other drugs, she cannot expect to adjust to being substance free in a few days.

Acquiring information about the disorders, the role of professional therapy, the role of medications, and the role of self-help programs in ongoing recovery is an essential component of this phase. The client learns about her diagnoses, causes and effects of dual disorders, and treatment. Information can empower, motivate, and help her learn how to change.

In this phase of recovery, the client learns to manage cravings to use alcohol or drugs and learns symptoms of the psychiatric illness. The client gets involved in self-help programs such as (1) AA, NA, CA, Women for Sobriety (WFS), Rational Recovery (RR) for the addiction; (2) Double Trouble, MISA, SAMI, CAMI, or Dual Recovery Anonymous (DRA) programs for dual disorders; (3) Emotions Anonymous (EA), Recovery, Inc., for any type of emotional problem; or (4) mental support groups for specific psychiatric illnesses (i.e., anxiety disorder support groups, manic-depression support groups). Decisions about which support groups to attend should be made by the client and treatment team.

The client's motivation gets stronger as she learns there are many steps that can be taken to recover. She becomes more comfortable accepting help and support from professionals, sponsors and members of support programs, and family members.

A major aspect of this phase is accepting the need for long-term involvement in recovery. The client works closely with the counselor and treatment team in developing and prioritizing her problems and using problem-solving strategies to address select problems from this list. She accepts the need for abstinence from alcohol, street drugs, and non-prescribed drugs. There is recognition that substance use can interfere with psychiatric recovery, lead the client back to the primary drug of abuse, or cause another addiction. She becomes less preoccupied with alcohol and other drugs and learns to counteract euphoric recall or positive thoughts about substances.

The client's family should continue their involvement in treatment. The degree to which they are involved depends on the client's treatment needs, the family's treatment needs, and the recommendations of caregivers. Excluding the family from ongoing involvement in recovery can cause serious problems.

> *Case #1: Faye is a 59-year-old divorced unemployed mother of two daughters and one son. She sought treatment for chronic depression, chronic anxiety, family problems, and alcoholism. During the first four months of treatment, she canceled most outpatient sessions and continued to drink alcohol on a daily basis despite experiencing severe symptoms of depression and anxiety. When she finally accepted the fact that her alcohol use was a major factor in her inability to improve her anxiety and depression, she reluctantly agreed to enter the hospital for detoxification and medication evaluation. Once stabilized, Faye became involved in outpatient treatment and was able to focus both on staying sober and reducing her anxiety and depression.*

> *Case #2: Twanda is a 38-year-old single woman with a history of schizophrenia, alcoholism, and polysubstance abuse (pot, cocaine, and many pills). During periods of active use, Twanda decompensates and becomes psychotic. She stops taking psychiatric medications, stops attending partial hospital programming, and seldom keeps her appointments with her treatment team. Her condition recently worsened following six months of fairly stable functioning when she started drinking on a daily basis. Twanda did not stabilize until an involuntary commitment was initiated after she stopped eating and threatened to kill herself.*

Phase 3—Early Recovery

This phase involves continued work at recovery from the dual disorders. The client learns to manage cravings and desires to use. He avoids people, places, events, and things that represent a relapse risk for addiction. Since the client cannot avoid all risk factors, he learns strategies to resist pressures from others to use substances. He becomes more used to coping with the physical, emotional, and social adjustments of sobriety.

The client learns to challenge and change addictive thinking. The sober side takes a stronger role than the addicted side, and the client more openly embraces the need for a recovery program that accepts abstinence as the goal. He may still want to use substances, but understands and accepts this as a normal aspect of addiction. The client knows that he can cope with this addicted self by using the tools of recovery.

During early recovery, the client learns more strategies to manage the psychiatric disorder and the problems it caused in his life. He learns that while medication can help improve symptoms of the psychiatric illness, he has to work at making changes in himself and his lifestyle to achieve a more fulfilling recovery.

The client learns to challenge and change negative or inaccurate thinking that contributes to anxiety, depression, or unhappiness. He becomes more realistic about recovery and the need for active involvement in a program of change. There is an increased awareness of the role of biology, behaviors, thinking, and personality in the development and maintenance of the psychiatric disorder.

Early recovery involves building structure and regularity into daily life to keep busy, stay focused on recovery, and enjoy leisure activities. Structure helps the client focus on goals and serves as a protective factor against relapse.

In family sessions, the focus is on understanding the impact of the dual disorders on the family. Initially, this is difficult and exacerbates guilt and shame. Family sessions aid the family in learning how they can support the client's recovery and what they should not do. Both the client and family learn to communicate more openly. This work with the family helps set the stage for the client to make amends later in the recovery process.

Working with a sponsor, using the Twelve Steps and other "tools" of AA, NA, and DRA are important aspects of the change plan. As the client progresses through this phase, he feels less guilty and shameful and comes to see himself not as a "bad person," but as an "ill person." He accepts that support from others is needed because recovery is difficult and presents many challenges.

Early recovery roughly involves the three to six months after the stabilization phase. Similar to previous phases, some clients work through this phase more easily than others. If the client relapses to alcohol or drug use, or experiences a worsening of psychiatric symptoms during this phase, he will need to restabilize before the issues discussed above can be addressed in treatment.

> *Case #1: Janet is a 40-year-old married mother of two daughters. This is her second involvement in outpatient treatment for severe anxiety and panic symptoms, post-traumatic stress disorder, and drug addiction (tranquilizers and pot). During her first outpatient treatment, she never addressed her addiction and received limited benefit from medications and psychotherapy. Janet attends individual and group sessions and is seen with her family every several weeks. She takes medication for her anxiety and panic symptoms and is learning to cope with exacerbations of symptoms without constantly seeking medications. Janet is realizing that while medications can help, they can't alleviate all of her symptoms or problems and, there is no "magic bullet" for all that ails her. She attends AA meetings and spends time at a local recovery club. She's been able to cope with several "close calls" and social pressures to use drugs. When she feels close to using, she reminds herself that her daughters suffer when she gets high because Janet becomes irresponsible and spends most of her time away from home. Janet is working on changing her anxious, depressed, and angry thoughts. In family sessions, she is focusing on improving communication and controlling anger toward her mother.*

> *Case #2: Stan is a 20-year old college student diagnosed with schizotypal personality disorder, depression, alcohol dependence, and polysubstance abuse (primarily marijuana and PCP). He was hospitalized briefly following a psychotic episode. He has not used substances since discharged from the hospital five months ago, and is active in AA and outpatient therapy. He has shown moderate improvements in his depressive symptoms and is about 70 percent compliant in taking his antidepressant medications. Stan evidences considerable difficulties in setting goals for himself, structuring his time, and relating to other people. His main emphases in treatment thus far have been learning to socialize with others without using pot in order to fit in, adding structure to his days so that he doesn't spent most of his time watching TV alone, and coping with persistent feelings of depression. He attends NA and AA and has a sponsor. Stan's mood has improved modestly. He still complains of low motivation and poor interpersonal relationships but is beginning to explore ways to deal with these issues.*

Phase 4—Middle Recovery

In this phase, the client shares more about her inner thoughts and feelings and reaches a greater level of self-awareness. Therapeutic work is directed toward improving interpersonal relationships. This requires communicating more openly with others and nurturing relationships. She not only gets support and help from others, but also gives to others. This helps her maintain balanced relationships that are not one-sided.

The client repairs the damage to relationships caused by the dual disorders. Steps 8 and 9 of AA, NA, CA, or DRA are addressed with a sponsor or counselor. These steps help the client to identify others hurt by her behaviors, become willing to make amends, and figure out ways to make amends when doing so will not hurt others. Relationships become more satisfying as a result of this process. In relationships that cannot be repaired or salvaged, the client learns to accept this reality rather than judge herself harshly.

During this phase, the client uses her unique sense of spirituality to aid recovery and personal growth. This process may or may not involve participation in formal religion. Many clients find strength and hope in attending religious services and praying.

Coping strategies strengthen as the client practices new ways of thinking, feeling, and behaving. As positive changes are made, the client feels less demoralized by the dual disorders. This enables her to stop blaming society, bad breaks, bad genes, or others for her problems.

Because addictive and psychiatric disorders are often chronic relapsing illnesses, the client learns to identify and manage warning signs of relapse. She learns that going back to using alcohol and drugs does not usually "come out of the blue," but represents a movement away from recovery toward relapse over a period of time. Similarly, the client learns that new episodes of psychiatric illness or significant worsening of persistent and chronic psychiatric symptoms often occur gradually over time. Knowing potential relapse warning signs allows the client to develop strategies to reduce the likelihood of relapse to either disorder. By daily monitoring of recovery, the client is in a position to spot relapse warning signs early, which helps her take action before things get out of hand.

If the psychiatric illness was a first episode and the client is symptom free, she may be withdrawn from medications. Usually, this is not done until the client has been doing well for several months or longer. If the client has a recurrent psychiatric disorder or a chronic persistent form of illness such as schizophrenia or bipolar illness, she remains on medications, even if doing well. The purpose of medications is to maintain gains and "prevent" a recurrence of illness. It is still possible for symptoms to break through even if the client takes medications. However, this happens less often than when medications are stopped prematurely.

As the client progresses through this phase, the focus shifts toward becoming a better person and more satisfied with oneself. Steps 10 and 11 in particular help in this process.

Middle recovery involves the six- to twelve-month period following early recovery. As in other phases, some move through this phase more easily than others.

> *Case #1: Art is a single, 29-year-old college graduate with an obsessive-compulsive disorder (OCD) and alcoholism. His OCD became so severe that he became paralyzed at work and was unable to complete simple tasks. He eventually lost his job as a result. He finally sought psychiatric treatment at the recommendation of a friend. Art currently takes medications for his OCD, attends a partial hospital program, and attends AA meetings. His OCD symptoms have improved markedly, and Art has been sober for ten months. In treatment, he is focusing on improving communication and relationship skills. He has decreased his high expectations of others, is less critical of himself and others, and is more positive in his conversations. Art is also working on using the support of others and asking others for help.*

> *Case #2: Lois is a 52-year-old widowed mother of four in treatment for alcoholism and recurrent depression. She's had periods of sobriety up to three years and currently has been sober for one year. Lois has had multiple episodes of depression, several of which were precipitated by stopping medications or drinking alcohol. She currently takes antidepressants, attends outpatient sessions twice a month, and attends AA three to five times a week. In treatment, Lois is focusing on her patterns of alcohol relapse and recurrences of depression so she is more aware of early warning signs. Although comfortable with accepting her alcoholism as a chronic disease, she struggles with seeing the chronicity of her depressive illness. Lois is also focusing on developing her spirituality as she ignored this during previous attempts at recovery. She has a sponsor and, despite some difficulties opening up and sharing her situation, Lois is using her sponsor to help her through rough times. Her sponsor has helped Lois figure out ways to make amends to her adult children. Although this initially evoked guilt, Lois's relationships have improved with three of her children. She is more realistic and patient with her youngest daughter, who is still angry at her.*

Phase 5—Late Recovery

In this phase, the client explores personal issues in greater depth as a solid foundation for recovery has been established. The client focuses more on changing "character defects" and dealing with other problems caused by his personality style. He builds on personal strengths and works on changing weaknesses.

Late recovery involves working at finding greater meaning in life and developing more positive values. The spiritual and interpersonal aspects of recovery help the client in this quest for meaning. Recovery provides the client a chance to become a better and more fulfilled person. However, this only comes with patience, discipline, and hard work.

If the client is still in therapy, focus may shift toward greater self-exploration so the client better understands his defenses, personality style, patterns of behavior, values, strengths, and vulnerabilities. The client gains greater clarity on how his past influences current behavior.

The client is more able to focus on healing from emotional wounds related to growing up in a family where an addiction or mental health problem existed or other traumatic experiences such as incest or other forms of abuse. The client learns to face pain head-on rather than use it as a reason to use substances or as a reason not to make changes. He learns to let go of anger, disappointment, sadness, and hate. He learns to forgive others who have caused physical or emotional harm. If the client is unable to forgive, he lives with the pain and anger in ways that are not self-destructive.

In some instances, this healing occurs by working the Twelve Step program of AA, NA, or DRA. In other cases, it involves deeper exploration in therapy sessions. Therapy helps the client work through emotional pain and put the past in perspective. To aid healing, the client may also participate in Adult Children, Incest Survivors, or Codependency mutual support groups.

This phase provides an opportunity to "balance" recovery, work, love, relationships, fun, and spirituality. This phase involves one to two years after the middle recovery period.

> *Case #1: John is a 28-year-old employed married man with a history of depression starting during his teenage years. His alcohol and drug use worsened considerably, so he entered a rehabilitation program and joined AA. John had been sober for more than a year when he sought outpatient help for an episode of depression. He benefited from a trial of medications but is now medication free. He initially attended sessions weekly but now attends monthly. In treatment, once his mood was stabilized, John focused on coming to grips with his negative feelings toward his parents, especially his father. John also addressed what he called his "self-centeredness" after his wife became pregnant and he became aware of feeling deeply jealous and worried about not being the "center" of her attention. His initial negative feelings about fatherhood made him realize that he had to address some of his personality issues that he avoided because of his previous perception that he had no serious flaws to change. John also realized that he had to be more responsible economically and began looking at ways to handle money better now that he was going to have a child to support. He grew up in a wealthy family and developed very poor money management habits over the years. John has gradually learned to focus less on himself and more on his pregnant wife.*

> *Case #2: Liz is a 42-year-old single unemployed woman with borderline personality disorder, depression with psychotic features, and alcoholism. She has been in and out of mental health and addiction treatment programs since she was a teen as a result of suicide attempts, severe depression, and psychotic decompensations. After more than a year of good sobriety, she began focusing on sexual abuse issues from the past in therapy sessions and by joining an incest survivor's support group. Several weeks later, she became depressed and suicidal after being flooded by awful memories and feelings of intense rage. However, unlike previous times when attempting to deal with her past, Liz was able to appropriately use her therapist, AA sponsor, and support system and dealt with this crisis without getting drunk or entering the psychiatric hospital. These were significant achievements for her. Liz is also learning to rely less on her therapist and more on her social support system during crises. Whereas in the past, she expected her therapist to virtually be on call all the time to help with her frequent crises. Her ability to tolerate distress and negative affect has improved considerably. She is less judgmental toward herself and less prone to exaggerating her character flaws at the expense of ignoring her strengths and achievements.*

Phase 6—Maintenance

This phase involves continued work on the "self." The client shifts toward more self-reliance and relies less on others. The client still depends on others, but she is more capable of using inner resources to cope with thoughts, feelings, and problems in life.

Part of continued growth and development may come from "giving away" what was learned in recovery by sponsoring others and working Step 12. Some clients are able to use their experience, hope, and strength to help others in recovery through sponsorship.

Since the client is well-grounded in recovery, she is better able to deal with daily life problems. These problems are faced head-on. Coping with problems and changes in life are not as overwhelming as they were in the earlier phases of recovery.

The client uses mistakes to learn rather than as a reason to put herself down. She becomes more accepting of her limitations, weaknesses, and flaws. Goals are modified whenever they cannot be reached or are unrealistic.

Many illnesses are lifelong conditions. Therefore, during the maintenance phase, if the client has a recurrent or persistent form of psychiatric illness, she continues taking medications. By this phase, the client is "living the program" of recovery and continues to grow as an individual.

Case #1: Joan is a 36-year-old married mother of two sons who sought help for alcoholism and agoraphobia with panic attacks after many years of being virtually symptom free and sober. She called five treatment programs before finding one that agreed to treat her. By the time she sought treatment, she had lost her job and had immense trouble leaving her house except for essentials, such as shopping for groceries. Due to her high level of alcohol use and prior history of severe withdrawal symptoms, Joan was detoxified and stabilized on psychiatric medications. She then participated in regular outpatient sessions and AA meetings and continued taking medications. Following a year of stable recovery, Joan had an alcohol use relapse that lasted two weeks. Fortunately, she cut this relapse off quickly and suffered minimal damage in her life. Joan has now been doing very well for over two years and is seen every three months by her therapist and treatment team for medication checks. She has returned to work, is able to leave home whenever she wants, and seldom experiences any symptoms of her illness. Joan attends AA once or twice a week and feels comfortable coping with the infrequent desire to drink alcohol.

> *Case #2: Patrick is a 27-year-old married father of two who initially sought help for cocaine addiction and completed a rehabilitation program. About one year after being drug free, he became depressed and felt vulnerable to using drugs again so he sought outpatient treatment. Because he saw serious problems in his marriage as a factor in his depression, Patrick was seen in both individual and marital sessions. His marriage improved as he and his wife, also in recovery from addiction, learned to face their conflicts head-on and accept each other's differences and flaws. Patrick has been clean for more than four years and now sponsors three other men in NA. He is using the principles and tools of the Twelve Step program in his daily life. After being out of treatment for almost two years, Patrick sought short-term help for recurrent marital conflict. Patrick and his wife were able to use the sessions to improve their relationship. He continues to use his sponsor and the NA program to grow as an individual.*

As the case examples in this chapter show, clients face different issues and challenges during various phases of recovery. Recovery is not a linear process where one moves easily from one phase to another. Rather, issues overlap between phases and clients often experience crises, problems, and setbacks. They may move back and forth between phases of recovery. Some clients will not be interested in certain issues, such as changing character defects or developing spirituality. Others will not use Twelve Step programs, sponsors, or other support groups. Clinicians must be realistic about the degree of influence that can be exerted. While the "ideal" is for clients to address physical, psychological, interpersonal, family, and spiritual issues, the "reality" is that clinicians can work with the client where she is and must be careful about "pushing" recovery too hard. Many clients make positive changes even if they do not address all of the issues that clinicians feel are important. This chart summarizes phases of treatment, possible therapeutic issues and interventions, and criteria for client progress.

Phase of Treatment	Possible Therapeutic Issues	Possible Therapeutic Interventions	Criteria for Progress
1) *Transition and Engagement* (weeks or longer)	Establishing diagnoses Resistance of client Ambivalence/denial Acute symptoms of illnesses	Conduct assessment Review effects of disorders Involve family Validate ambivalence Provide motivational counseling Educate about illness and recovery Facilitate referrals Medication evaluation Provide support Introduce Twelve Steps	Acknowledges there is a problem with alcohol or drugs Acknowledges there is a mental health problem Agrees to participate in treatment Agrees to participate in self-help programs Stops or reduces substance use
2) *Stabilization* (weeks or longer)	Acute symptoms of illness Denial/minimization/grief Cravings/close calls Need for family and social support	Detoxification/medication Review dual-diagnosis history Monitor cravings and psychiatric symptoms Develop problem list Craving management Continue work on Twelve Steps Family sessions as needed	Accepts dual disorders; increased motivation Feels hopeful about recovery System is alcohol/drug free and withdrawal is over; or there aren't any more acute withdrawal symptoms Decrease in cravings and preoccupation with using Psychiatric symptoms don't seriously impair ability to function
3) *Early Recovery* (three to six months after Stabilization)	People, places, events, and things Negative feelings Guilt and shame Persistent psychiatric symptoms Impact on family Negative thinking Need for structure Lapse, relapse, and recurrences	Identify triggers and coping strategies Discuss negative feelings and coping strategies (anger, guilt, etc.) Identify and challenge cognitive distortions and other forms of negative thinking ("stinking" thinking) Leisure counseling Relapse prevention counseling Family sessions as needed Continue work on Twelve Steps	Feels less guilty and shameful Understanding of disorders (causes, effects, recovery issues, treatment strategies) Ability to cope with people, places, events, and things Management of feelings and psychiatric symptoms Active involvement in treatment and self help Connects with a support system and/or sponsor Deals with setbacks; accepts steps toward progress

Phase of Treatment	Possible Therapeutic Issues	Possible Therapeutic Interventions	Criteria for Progress
4) Middle Recovery (6–12 months after Early Recovery)	Interpersonal relationships Making amends Upsetting feelings Negative thinking Lapse, relapse, and recurrences Spirituality	Discuss ways to improve relationships and communications Make amends Continue practicing new ways of thinking Relapse education on warning signs and high-risk factors Relapse analysis Daily inventory Discuss spirituality issues May stop medications (for single episode of psychiatric illness) Family sessions as needed Continue work on Twelve Steps	Feels better about self in relationships Improve relationships and communication Thinking is more positive and less critical or hopeless Able to spot early warning signs of relapse Able to recover from lapse, relapse, or recurrence Increased comfort with spiritual aspect of recovery Less reliance on therapist or sponsor
5) Late Recovery (1+ years after Middle Recovery)	Continue work from previous phase Healing from emotional wounds of past Confront vs. avoid pain and conflict Forgiveness of others Sponsorship Lifestyle balance (work, play, love, recovery, spirituality, etc.) Personality (character defects)	Discuss ways to enhance meaning in life Reevaluate past experiences to reduce hurt and pain, and forgive others Discuss strategies to identify and face current emotional pain Focus on ways to balance major areas of life Discuss personality traits and strategies to change defects Continue work on Twelve Steps	Increase in self-exploration in treatment or with sponsor Increase in self-esteem and confidence Increase in feelings of serenity and satisfaction with life Increase in concern toward others "Gives back" to others through sponsorship and service Less reliant on others and more self-reliant Comfortable with personal strengths and weaknesses Uses the "tools" and "principles" of recovery in daily life
6) Maintenance	Continue work from previous phase Focuses on new problems and issues	Focus on continued "growth" Self-improvement	More balanced and satisfying life Tries to improve self (character, values, goals, coping strategies) and interpersonal relationships "Lives" the program in daily life

Chapter 3
Format of DDRC

Modalities of Treatment and Treatment Settings

Dual Disorders Recovery Counseling (DDRC) can be used in individual, family, and group sessions. This model can be used throughout the continuum of care in inpatient, residential, partial hospital, and outpatient settings. DDRC can be adapted and used in addiction treatment settings provided that appropriate training, supervision, and consultation are available for the counselor in relation to psychiatric issues.

Duration of Treatment

With changes brought about by managed care, the trend in treatment is moving away from inpatient care except in the most serious cases of acute illness. Treatments are getting shorter in length, requiring clinicians to limit specific issues and problems addressed. The DDRC model provides a framework and structure that can help clinicians adjust to the changing demands of managed care.

Acute inpatient dual diagnosis treatment usually lasts a week or so. Residential treatment programs may last several weeks or months. Partial hospitalization and intensive outpatient programs last two to eight weeks. Outpatient treatment lasts three to six months or longer. Recurrent conditions (major depression and bipolar illness) and persistent disorders (schizophrenia) require ongoing participation in maintenance pharmacotherapy and supportive counseling.

Compatibility with Other Treatments

DDRC is compatible with pharmacotherapy and family treatment. Many clients require medication to treat psychiatric symptoms or addiction in addition to therapy or counseling.[1] Therefore, medication compliance, the perception of taking medications as a recovering person, and potential adverse effects of alcohol or other drugs on medication efficacy are important issues to discuss.

Family participation in assessment and treatment is viewed as important and compatible with the DDRC model. The family can:

1. Provide important information in the assessment process.
2. Provide support to the recovering client.
3. Help identify early signs of addiction relapse or psychiatric recurrence and point these out to the recovering dual diagnosed family member.
4. Address their questions, concerns, and reactions to the disorders.
5. Address their own problems and issues.

A combination of family psychoeducational, counseling, and support programs can be used. Referrals for assessment of serious problems (psychiatric, substance abuse, behavioral) among specific family members can also be initiated as necessary (i.e., a child of a client who is suicidal, depressed, or getting in trouble at school can be referred for a psychiatric evaluation and treatment).

Role of Mutual Support Programs

All clients are educated regarding self-help programs and linked with specific programs when appropriate. The self-help programs recommended may include AA, NA, CA, and other addiction support groups such as Rational Recovery, SMART Recovery, or Women for Sobriety; Dual Recovery Anonymous, Double Trouble, and other dual recovery support groups, and mental health support groups. Sponsorship, literature, slogans, and recovery clubs are helpful in recovery. However, DDRC does not assume that a client cannot recover without involvement in a Twelve Step group or that failure to attend Twelve Step groups is a sign of "resistance." Clients may use "tools" of programs even if meetings are not attended.

Clients Best Suited for This Counseling Approach

DDRC can be adapted for any type or combination of dual disorders. However, it is best suited for mood, anxiety, psychotic, personality, adjustment, and other addictive disorders in combination with a substance use disorder.

Clients with mental retardation, organic brain syndromes, head injuries, and more severe forms of thought disorders are less suited for this counseling approach. However, many individuals with psychotic disorders can benefit from DDRC.

Counselor's Role

As evidenced by the list of counselor behaviors in Chapter 4, many roles are assumed by the clinician: educator, collaborator, adviser, advocate, and problem solver.

Although the counselor is active asking questions, clarifying problems and feelings, and helping the client learn strategies to cope with problems, the client talks the most during individual DDRC sessions. In psychoeducational groups, the counselor is active in providing education to the group. Clients are encouraged to ask questions, share personal experiences, and express their ideas on ways to cope with problems or recovery issues reviewed during the group session. In therapy or problem-solving groups, the group leader is less active verbally than in psychoeducational groups.

Directiveness of Counselor

In DDRC, the counselor may be directive and active with one client and less directive and active with another. The approach must be individualized and take into account each client's strengths, abilities, deficits, and response to feedback. However, the counselor is generally more directive than in traditional mental health counseling, particularly in relation to continued substance use, relapse setups, pointing out self-defeating behavior patterns, recommending support group meetings, and pointing out concrete strategies for handling alcohol or drug cravings, pressures to use, or ways to deal with negative affect or interpersonal conflict. Advice is given after eliciting the client's ideas on coping strategies for particular problems.

Therapeutic Alliance (TA)

A TA facilitates recovery[2] and is based on the counselor's ability to "connect with the client," respect differences, show empathy, use humor, and understand the "inner world" of the client. Listening; providing information; being supportive, encouraging, and humorous; and being up front and directive can help build the TA.

A poor alliance may show in missed appointments or failure to comply with treatment. Discussing common problems in recovery and acknowledging specific problems between the counselor and client can improve the TA. Calling clients who drop out of treatment early and inquiring as to whether they think a new treatment plan can help may help correct a poor TA. Discussion of specific cases in supervision can help the counselor identify causes of a poor TA and strategies to correct it.

Chapter 4
Counselor Training and Supervision

Content Areas for Training

The counselor needs to have a broad knowledge of assessment and treatment of dual disorders. Specific areas with which the counselor should be familiar include:

1. Psychiatric illnesses: types, causes, symptoms, and effects.
2. Substance use disorders: types and effects of substances, causes, symptoms, and effects of SUDs.
3. The relationships between the psychiatric and substance use disorders.
4. Integrated treatment strategies for dual disorders, how to develop a group program, and the importance of a therapeutic milieu in inpatient or residential settings.
5. Psychosocial treatment approaches for various disorders (i.e., treatments for PTSD, obsessive-compulsive disorder, motivational enhancement therapy for substance use disorders).
6. Somatic treatments: medications for both types of disorders and electroshock therapy for certain mental disorders.
7. Self-help programs for substance use, psychiatric, and dual disorders.
8. Family issues in treatment and recovery.
9. Strategies to enhance motivation and improve treatment adherence.
10. The recovery process and phases of recovery.
11. The continuum of care for both addiction and psychiatric illnesses and local community resources.
12. Relapse precipitants, warning signs, and relapse prevention strategies for both disorders.
13. Dealing with crises and emergencies: suicidality, relapse, and the process of involuntary hospitalization.
14. Strategies to deal with refractory or treatment resistant clients with recurrent or chronic forms of mental illness.
15. How to use bibliotherapeutic and behavioral assignments to facilitate recovery.

The counselor must be able to develop a therapeutic alliance with clients who have differing abilities to utilize treatment. This requires awareness of one's owns issues, biases, limitations, and strengths and a willingness to examine reactions to clients.

The counselor needs to network with case managers of other service providers because many dual diagnosis clients have multiple psychosocial needs and problems. Since crises may arise, the counselor must also be conversant with crisis intervention approaches. An ability to work with a team is also essential in all treatment contexts.

Experience with substance abusing and mental health clients is the ideal. However, if a counselor is trained in one field and has access to additional training and supervision in the other, it is possible to expand knowledge and skills and work effectively with dual diagnosed clients.

Counselor's Recovery Status and Attitudes

If a counselor has the training, knowledge, and experiential background in working with psychiatric clients and those with substance use disorders, a personal history of recovery can be helpful. Although self-disclosure is sometimes appropriate, the counselor shares less of his own recovery experience than typically is shared in the more traditional addiction treatment settings.

Helpful attitudes and characteristics of counselors include: hope and optimism for recovery, a high degree of empathy, patience and tolerance, flexibility, an ability to enjoy working with difficult clients, a realistic perspective on change and steps toward success, a low need to control the client, an ability to engage the client yet be able to detach, and an ability to utilize a multiplicity of treatment interventions rather than relying on a single way of counseling.

Counselor's Behaviors

The DDRC approach involves a broad range of behaviors and interventions of the counselor. Specific behaviors depend on the severity of the client's symptoms, his related needs and problems, and the treatment contract. Interventions include the following:

1. Providing information and education.
2. Providing support and encouragement.
3. Challenging denial and self-destructive behaviors. Confrontation is modified to take into account the client's ego strength and ability to tolerate confrontation.
4. Providing feedback on problems and progress in treatment.
5. Encouraging and monitoring abstinence from alcohol, illicit drugs, and non-prescribed drugs.
6. Facilitating involvement in self-help groups.
7. Helping the client identify, prioritize, and work on specific problems.
8. Monitoring addiction recovery issues (cravings, close calls, people, places, events, and things, and high-risk relapse factors).
9. Monitoring target psychiatric symptoms (suicidality, mood symptoms, anxiety symptoms, psychotic symptoms, or problem behaviors).

10. Helping the client develop specific recovery skills (i.e., coping with cravings, refusing offers to get high, challenging faulty thinking, coping with negative affect, improving interpersonal behaviors).

11. Developing relapse prevention strategies.

12. Facilitating inpatient admissions when needed.

13. Facilitating the use of community resources or services.

14. Advocating on behalf of the client.

15. Developing therapeutic assignments aimed at helping the client reach a goal or make a specific change.

16. Following up when a client fails to follow through with treatment in order to offer support, crisis intervention, and outreach.

Counselor's Behaviors Contraindicated

The counselor does not interpret the client's behaviors or motivation. The focus is more on understanding and coping with issues related to the dual disorders and current functioning. The counselor avoids extensive exploration of past traumas during the early phases of recovery because this can lead to avoidance of addressing the substance use disorder, and it can increase the client's anxiety. Harsh confrontation is avoided because this can adversely impact the client's sense of self. Moreover, it can drive the client away from treatment. Confrontation is used, but should be done in a caring, nonjudgmental, nonpunitive, and reality-oriented manner.

Supervision

Supervision provides counselors an opportunity to develop and improve knowledge and skills. It provides a mechanism to address their clinical concerns and personal reactions to clients, thus allowing them to work through unhelpful attitudes, feelings, or behaviors that impede the counseling process. Supervision also provides a mechanism for accountability so that the counselor's work can be monitored for "quality of care" and other administrative reasons to insure productivity requirements are being met. Supervision can help the counselor:

1. Increase knowledge of dual disorders and the counseling process.

2. Improve specific counseling skills (i.e., setting an agenda, helping client develop new coping skills, using motivational interventions).

3. Deal with personal issues or reactions that impede therapeutic alliance or progress (i.e., anger toward a client who relapses, negative reactions to a client with a personality disorder).

4. Use personal strengths in the counseling process (i.e., use of own experiences, use of humor).

5. Maintain a balanced therapeutic focus on the client's substance use and mental health disorders.
6. Figure out strategies to work through impasses in treatment.

Formats for Supervision

A variety of formats can be used for supervision. The less knowledgeable and experienced a counselor is, the more extensive the supervision should be. Supervision should not solely focus on routine review of cases but more on in-depth discussions of difficult clinical cases or areas in which the counselor wants to improve. Formats for supervision include:

1. Discussion of individual cases, family sessions, or group treatment sessions.
2. Review of written assessments, clinical notes, and treatment plans.
3. Live observation of counseling sessions.
4. Review and discussion of audiotapes or videotapes of counseling sessions.
5. Conducting co-therapy sessions.
6. Group supervision with other counselors in which individual, family, or groups are reviewed, and clinical concerns of mutual interest are shared and explored.

The most helpful but time intensive formats are those where the counselor can be observed conducting a session. This provides opportunities to identify personal or professional areas needing further attention. This is especially helpful for less experienced counselors. Once a counselor works through anxiety about being scrutinized in vivo or on tape, he usually finds this process helpful for professional development.

Counselors should receive specific feedback regarding their work. This includes reinforcement for good work and critical feedback on areas of weakness. For example, a group counselor can benefit from feedback pointing out that he talks too much in the group sessions or tells clients how to cope with a recovery issue before eliciting their ideas on coping strategies. Similarly, counselors need to hear positive feedback on what they do well in treatment sessions.

Use of Adherence Scales

The use of adherence scales, which are routinely used in clinical research, is an excellent way to provide feedback on treatment sessions. The counselor is rated on performing specific interventions and the quality of these interventions. The major drawback is that tapes of treatment sessions have to be reviewed in detail, a process requiring considerable time. This process is helpful to newer, less-experienced counselors although all clinicians can benefit from feedback regarding their work.

The following are sample adherence scales that can be used in rating individual and group treatment sessions. These scales are modeled after ones we used in clinical research projects.

Adherence Scale for Dual Disorders Recovery Counseling Individual Treatment Sessions

Counselor: _____ Rater: _____

Session Date: _____ Date Rated: _____

Date Reviewed with Counselor: _____

Rate the quality of the counselor's interventions (i.e., how helpful and appropriate were the counselor's interventions during the session) using the seven-point rating scale below. Mark your rating in the blank to the immediate left of each item.

1	2	3	4	5	6	7
Not at all		Some		Considerably		Very much

Quality   Supporting Recovery and Motivating Client

_____ 1. Encouraging client to set an agenda for each counseling session.

_____ 2. Encouraging client to discuss both the psychiatric and substance use problems.

_____ 3. Encouraging client to discuss close calls and cravings for drugs or alcohol and ways to manage them.

_____ 4. Encouraging client to accept abstinence from alcohol, street drugs, and non-prescribed medications as a recovery goal.

_____ 5. Encouraging client to focus on problem solving and identifying positive coping strategies related to specific issues or problems discussed.

_____ 6. Encouraging client to discuss any substance use or significant change in psychiatric symptoms.

_____ 7. Limiting discussions in counseling sessions to one or two problem areas.

_____ 8. Assigning therapeutic tasks to be completed between treatment sessions (i.e., completion of workbook activity, reading chapter of AA Big Book, NA Basic Text, Dual Recovery Book).

_____ 9. Reviewing completed assignments in treatment sessions. If client failed to complete an assignment, discussing the reasons.

Quality	Providing Feedback
_____ 1.	Discussing denial of client.
_____ 2.	Pointing out self-defeating behaviors on the part of the client.
_____ 3.	Helping client discuss the adverse effects of self-defeating behaviors, both on self and others.
_____ 4.	Pointing out strengths of client and providing reinforcement for positive behaviors and coping strategies used.
_____ 5.	Helping the client understand the connection between thoughts, feelings, and behaviors.

Quality	Providing Information and Education
_____ 1.	Educating client about psychiatric illness, addiction, and the relationship between dual disorders.
_____ 2.	Helping client relate to educational material in a personal way (i.e., when discussing relapse warning signs, have client give personal examples of warning signs).
_____ 3.	Educating client about treatments for dual disorders (professional therapies, medications, and self-help programs).
_____ 4.	Providing client with information on specific issues or problems pertinent to his situation (i.e., depression, anger, NA, relapse, family issues in medications).

Quality	Encouraging Participation in Self-Help Programs
_____ 1.	Encouraging participation in Twelve Step groups, mental health support groups, and/or dual recovery groups.
_____ 2.	Expressing positive opinions about support groups.
_____ 3.	Encouraging client to get and use an NA/AA/CA/DRA sponsor for help and support during recovery.
_____ 4.	Discussing resistances or negative views that client has regarding self-help programs or sponsors.

Quality	Discharge Planning (for Inpatients)
_____ 1.	Encouraging client to participate in ongoing professional treatment (partial hospital program, outpatient therapy).
_____ 2.	Identifying barriers to follow-up treatment after hospital discharge.

_____ 3. Helping client identify positive aspects of continued treatment.

_____ 4. Encouraging client to participate in self-help programs, use a sponsor, and get a "home group."

_____ 5. Helping client identify specific problems and treatment issues to focus on in ongoing outpatient treatment.

_____ 6. Helping client understand the connection between ongoing involvement in therapy and self-help programs and positive treatment outcome.

_____ 7. Helping client develop an "emergency plan" to deal with suicidal risk or unexpected setbacks or relapses to either disorder.

Adherence Scale for Dual Disorders Recovery Counseling Group Treatment Sessions

Counselor: _____ Rater: _____

Type of Group: ___Psychoeducational   ___Problem Solving   ___Therapy   ___Family

Session Topic (for Psychoeducational Group): _____

Session Date: _____ Date Rated: _____

Date Reviewed with Counselor: _____

Rate the quality of the counselor's interventions (i.e., how helpful and appropriate were the counselor's interventions during the group session) using the seven-point rating scale below. Mark your rating in the blank to the immediate left of each item.

1	2	3	4	5	6	7
Not at all		Some		Considerably		Very much

Quality   Supporting Recovery and Motivating Client

_____ 1. Encouraging clients to discuss both the psychiatric and substance use problems.

_____ 2. Encouraging clients to discuss cravings for drugs or alcohol or "close calls."

_____ 3. Encouraging clients to discuss any episodes of actual substance use and strategies to stop use.

_____ 4. Encouraging clients to accept abstinence from alcohol, street drugs, and non-prescribed medications as a recovery goal.

_____ 5. Encouraging clients to discuss both behavioral and cognitive coping strategies related to specific recovery issues or problems discussed.

_____ 6. Encouraging clients to discuss psychiatric problems and coping strategies.

Quality   Providing Feedback

_____ 1. Discussing the denial of a client or encouraging other group members to do so.

_____ 2. Pointing out self-defeating behaviors of clients or encouraging other group members to do so.

_____ 3. Helping clients discuss the adverse effects of self-defeating behaviors, both on self and others.

_____ 4. Pointing out strengths of clients and providing reinforcement for positive behaviors or coping strategies used.

_____ 5. Helping clients understand the connection between thoughts, feelings, and behaviors.

Quality — Providing Information and Education

_____ 1. Educating clients about psychiatric illness, addiction, and relationships between dual disorders.

_____ 2. Helping clients relate to psychoeducational material in a personal way.

_____ 3. Educating clients about treatments for dual disorders (professional therapies, medications, and self-help programs).

_____ 4. Educating clients about the role of medication in recovery from psychiatric illness and effects of using alcohol or drugs on efficacy of medications.

_____ 5. Providing clients with information on specific issues or problems pertinent to their situation (i.e., information on depression, anger, AA or NA, relapse, family issues in recovery, antidepressant medications).

Quality — Encouraging Participation in Self-Help Programs

_____ 1. Encouraging participation in Twelve Step groups, mental health support groups, and/or dual recovery groups.

_____ 2. Expressing positive opinions about support groups.

_____ 3. Encouraging clients to get and use an NA/AA/CA/DRA sponsor.

_____ 4. Discussing resistances or negative views that clients have regarding self-help programs or sponsors.

Quality — Facilitating Group Participation

_____ 1. Encouraging all clients to participate in group discussions.

_____ 2. Encouraging clients to give one another constructive feedback.

_____ 3. Encouraging clients to be specific when discussing strategies to cope with recovery issues or problems related to either disorder.

_____ 4. Encouraging clients to discuss recovery plans they will occur between group sessions.

_____ 5. Ensuring that one or two clients don't dominate the entire group discussion so all members talk in the session.

Quality   For Psychoeducational Groups

_____ 1. Educating clients on group topic by reviewing major points identified in the session outline.

_____ 2. Encouraging clients to relate to psychoeducational material by sharing personal experiences or reactions.

_____ 3. Facilitating discussion among clients of their responses to the group session psychoeducational material.

_____ 4. Keeping discussions focused on the session topic.

Quality   For Problem-Solving Groups

_____ 1. Helping clients identify and prioritize specific concerns and problems to discuss in the group session.

_____ 2. Facilitating discussion among clients of various problems and concerns presented.

_____ 3. Helping clients identify and discuss strategies to cope with the various problems or concerns identified (ensuring adequate time is spent on coping strategies, not just discussion of problems).

_____ 4. Keeping discussions focused on problems and concerns raised by clients in the group.

Chapter 5
The Assessment Process

Components of Assessment

The initial assessment involves a combination of the following: psychiatric evaluation, mental status exam, substance use history, physical examination, laboratory work, and urinalysis. Client and collateral interviews and review of previous records can be part of the process.

Ongoing assessment involves monitoring psychiatric symptoms and substance use. Questions asked during counseling sessions, discussions with family or other service providers, completion of rating scales, blood work (for clients on certain medications), urine drug screens, and breathalyzer tests can be used to continuously assess the client.

Assessment should also address the client's strengths and resiliencies. All clients have personal strengths that can aid them in recovery. Many are resilient and have bounced back from relapses or major life problems.

American Psychiatric Association (APA) DSM Classification

A comprehensive assessment reviews information on all areas of functioning of the client: reason for seeking help and current stressors; current and past psychiatric symptoms (including suicidality and homicidality); current and past substance use; history of treatment and relapse; medical, family, social, developmental, academic, occupational, legal, and spiritual history; and mental status examination.

The substance use history includes a detailed review of current and past substances used (frequency, quantity, methods of use) and effects of such use on psychiatric symptoms. It reviews DSM symptoms of substance use disorders such as: loss of control; inability to abstain despite repeated attempts; obsession or preoccupation with using, getting, or recovering from the effects of substances; significant increase or decrease in tolerance; withdrawal symptoms or using to avoid these symptoms; continued substance use despite problems; and impairment caused by substance use.

Clinical diagnoses are formulated based on criteria set forth by the APA's *Diagnostic and Statistical Manual of Mental Disorders*.[1] The DSM-IV TR provides a comprehensive approach to assessment of the client, which is recorded on five axes:

1. *Axis I: clinical disorders.* These include schizophrenia and other psychotic disorders; mood, anxiety, somatoform, factitious, dissociative, sexual and gender identity disorders; eating, sleep, impulse control, and adjustment disorders. Each specific disorder has a cluster of physical, emotional, behavioral, or cognitive symptoms, time requirements, and functioning impairments associated with it. If it is hard to determine if a disorder exists but the client manifests symptoms of it, a rule-out diagnosis can be given while additional observations are made over time.

2. *Axis II: personality disorders and mental retardation.* These include paranoid, schizoid, schizotypal, antisocial, borderline, histrionic, narcissistic, avoidant, dependent, obsessive-compulsive, and personality disorder not otherwise specified. Even if the client does not meet full criteria for a personality disorder, the clinician can note significant "traits" on Axis II (e.g., antisocial, narcissistic, paranoid). Axis II disorders, especially antisocial and borderline disorders, are common among clients with Axis I disorders and often complicate recovery.

3. *Axis III: general medical conditions and disorders.* These include any condition, disorder, or disease caused by injury, poisoning, or infection; any disorders associated with pregnancy, childbirth, or the postpartum period; or a disorder involving the nervous system, blood, sense organs, skin, or any of the major systems (circulatory, respiratory, digestive, genitourinary, musculoskeletal). Substance use disorders are associated with increased risk of injury and diseases. Many clients enter treatment with significant medical problems in addition to their substance use and psychiatric disorders.

4. *Axis IV: psychosocial and environmental problems.* These include problems with the primary support group or social environment, education, occupation, housing, economic status, access to health care, crime, and related to the legal system. These problems may contribute to the exacerbation of the current disorder or result from it. Axis IV is also coded for severity (e.g., none, minimal, mild, moderate, severe, extreme). Many studies document high rates of psychosocial and environmental problems among clients with dual disorders.[2]

5. Axis V: Global assessment of functioning (current and past year). This is the clinician's judgment of the patient's current overall level of functioning and highest level of functioning within the past year related to interpersonal relationships, occupation, and use of leisure time. Level of functioning includes superior, very good, good, fair, poor, very poor, and grossly impaired.

American Society on Addiction Medicine Framework (ASAM)

Clinical interviews can review the ASAM criteria below and may use the Addiction Severity Index or other interview formats, as well as pen and pencil questionnaires such as the Michigan Alcoholism Screen Test (MAST), the Drug Abuse Screening Test (DAST), or the Dartmouth Assessment of Lifestyle Inventory (DALI), which is one of the only questionnaires designed for clients with dual disorders. Breathalyzers, urine and blood tests, liver function studies, and a physical examination can also aid the assessment process.

ASAM delineates the following six dimensions of functioning to assess the level of care needed for the client:[3]

1. *Acute intoxication and withdrawal potential.* This determines if the client needs medical detoxification prior to initiating another type of treatment. An important issue is facilitating the client's linkage into continued treatment or self-help recovery following detoxification.

2. *Biomedical conditions and complications.* This determines the level of medical management required for the client with acute or chronic medical problems.
3. *Emotional, behavioral, or cognitive conditions and complications.* This determines whether the client has a co-occurring psychiatric illness or other significant symptoms requiring treatment, and whether treatment in a mental health system is needed for recurrent or persistent forms of mental disorders.
4. *Readiness to change.* This determines level of motivation of the client to change, and the degree to which treatment recommendations are accepted or resisted.
5. *Relapse, continued use, or continued problem potential.* This determines whether the client is aware of relapse triggers and has a plan or needs to stabilize from a recent relapse. This dimension also aims to assess whether the client is suicidal or has mental health problems that may impede his ability to engage in treatment.
6. *Recovery/living environment.* This determines if other people, school, work, child care or transportation problems are a barrier to the client's ability to engage in treatment. It also helps assess the degree to which the client has a support system that can aid recovery.

The assessment findings are used to recommend a level of care: outpatient, intensive outpatient, partial hospital, medically monitored inpatient detoxification, short-term residential, long-term residential, or medically managed inpatient detoxification or residential care. Clients may be referred to a dual diagnosis "capable" or "enhanced" program. Dual diagnosis *capable* programs are offered in an addiction treatment system to treat less severely psychiatrically ill clients. They focus primarily on treatment of the substance use disorder among clients whose mental disorders are stable. Dual diagnosis *enhanced* programs are likely to be part of a mental health system of care. These programs care for clients with more unstable or disabling mental disorders in addition to the substance use disorder.

Assessment Instruments

Specific instruments may be used to gather objective and subjective data. These may be administered by a professional (e.g., SCID or personality disorder interviews). Or they may be completed by the client (e.g., Beck or Hamilton depression or anxiety inventories; mania scales or other scales for psychiatric disorders; or the MAST, DAST, or DALI for substance use problems).[4] These instruments can be used to gather baseline data and to measure change in symptoms over time. The American Psychiatric Association's *Handbook of Psychiatric Measures* provides descriptions of numerous scales that can be used during the baseline assessment and follow-up.[5]

Workbook Assignments

Review of recovery workbook assignments is also useful in assessing the client's problems, ability to develop recovery and change plans, or motivation to comply with treatment. Workbooks can be used by the counselor to identify specific areas of focus in individual or group DDRC sessions.

Quality Improvement (QI)

Assessing clients periodically is an excellent QI activity (also referred to as Performance Improvement Programs). This process provides important information on clients regarding how they function or change over time. QI data compiled on a clinic's client population provides information on a variety of important issues such as:

1. Changes in substance use.
2. Changes in psychiatric symptoms.
3. Relapse and rehospitalization rates.
4. Compliance with scheduled appointments with clinicians or doctors.
5. Medication compliance.
6. Client use of support groups.
7. Client use of other services (vocational, social service).
8. Rates of treatment completion.
9. Impact of dual disorders on the family.
10. Improvement in any area of psychosocial functioning.
11. Client or family satisfaction with services.

Chapter 6
Motivation and Treatment Adherence

Motivation and Treatment Readiness

Motivation to change affects treatment entry, adherence, and retention.[1] Motivational interventions have been shown to enhance treatment entry, retention, and completion rates among alcohol abusers,[2] opiate addicts,[3] and dual diagnosis clients with psychotic or mood disorders.[4] Assessing motivation or readiness to change helps clinicians "match" clients to clinical interventions.[5] For example, clients with low motivation may be better served by using strategies to enhance motivation rather than trying to implement a change plan before the client is ready.

Treatment Adherence, Retention, and Drop Out

Many studies of psychiatric disorders among substance abusers seeking treatment report an association with poor adherence and drop out from treatment and level of symptomatology,[6] particularly among clients with antisocial personality disorders[7] and those who attend standard substance abuse treatment programs rather than specialty dual diagnosis programs.[8] A review of seventeen studies addressing psychological problems found that the majority of studies show a positive correlation between high symptom levels at the time of admission and premature termination from treatment.[9]

One of our studies of discharged inpatients with depressive disorders and cocaine dependence participating in outpatient treatment found that clients receiving motivational therapy (MT) during the first month of outpatient care were more likely than those receiving usual care to complete thirty and ninety days of treatment. MT clients were also less likely to be rehospitalized within one year of entry into outpatient care.[10]

Medication Adherence

Medications help clients withdraw safely from addictive substances, cope with cravings, reduce the reinforcing properties of substances, maintain abstinence, and reduce relapse risk. Disulfiram and naltrexone are used with alcoholics to reduce cravings or desires to drink alcohol, create an aversive reaction when alcohol is ingested increasing the desire to avoid alcohol, and thus help to limit the intensity of relapses if the alcoholic resumes drinking.[11] Opiate antagonists such as naltrexone are used with drug addicts to block the euphoric effects of opiates and reduce the client's desire to use.[12]

Psychotropic medications are used to reduce symptoms and the risk of recurrence of psychiatric illness. However, many clients fail to accept the need for medications, fail to take them as prescribed, stop taking them prematurely, or take them in ways that pose health risks, such as ingesting alcohol or using illicit drugs with them.[13] Estimates of non-adherence with medication among psychotic clients are as high as 50 to 70 percent.[14]

Numerous factors contribute to poor adherence with medications. These include:
1. Uncomfortable side effects.
2. Unrealistic expectations of the purpose and efficacy of medicine.
3. Lack of adequate response to treatment.
4. Complicated medication regimes.
5. Negative interactions with alcohol or illicit drugs.
6. Low motivation to change.
7. Negative attitudes of clients regarding treatment.
8. Severity of illness.
9. Poor judgment.
10. In the case of substance abuse, the desire to use substances again.

Poor medication adherence increases the risk of relapse to substance abuse, psychiatric illness or both, and it contributes to rehospitalization. Among dual diagnosis clients, poor adherence with medication is associated with resumption of substance use and other problems in functioning.[15] Numerous studies of psychiatric rehospitalization show that clients who are readmitted, including high utilizers with multiple admissions, are significantly more likely to be noncompliant with psychotropic medications and significantly more likely to abuse alcohol or drugs.[16] Thus, medication adherence represents an important area in clinical care and the research evidence shows a strong association between poor adherence and negative clinical outcome. Clients who are poorly compliant with medications are often poorly compliant with aftercare or outpatient treatment sessions.

Adherence Enhancement Strategies

Strategies that have a positive impact on treatment adherence generally are in two categories:[17] (1) clinical strategies related to type, process, content and method of treatment, and (2) systems strategies related to how treatment services are organized and provided.

One set of clinical strategies relates to the clinician's attitudes and the relationship with the client. Adherence enhancing strategies include:
1. Focusing on the development of a therapeutic alliance with the client.
2. Identifying and addressing problems in the therapeutic alliance.
3. Conveying helpfulness in attitudes and behaviors (i.e., expressing empathy).

Another set of clinical strategies relates to the client's motivation or readiness to change, barriers that impede motivation, and preparing clients for moving from one level of care to another or preparing them for therapy. Clinical strategies improving adherence include:
1. Accepting and addressing the client's ambivalence regarding change.
2. Providing motivational interventions.

3. Preparing clients for psychotherapy (i.e., treatment induction).
4. Emphasizing that responsibility to change lies with the client.
5. Identifying potential barriers to change and ways to overcome these.
6. Negotiating rather than dictating treatment or change plans.

A final set of clinical strategies relates to type and intensity of treatment. Strategies associated with improved adherence include:

1. Helping clients with problems other than substance abuse or psychiatric illness.
2. Providing interventions based on empirical support.
3. Involving the client's family in treatment.
4. Providing aftercare adherence sessions prior to hospital discharge.
5. Helping the client cope with motivational roadblocks and relapse risk factors.
6. Offering incentives for adherence with treatment sessions or abstinence.
7. Facilitating the use of medications to reduce cravings for substances or control psychiatric symptoms.

Family and treatment systems related strategies that have a positive impact on adherence with treatment include the following:

1. Providing easy access to treatment in terms of location of services or prompt appointments when a client requests help.
2. Using phone calls or letters to remind clients of initial evaluation appointments, ongoing appointments, or outreach to clients who fail to show for appointments.
3. Developing a clinic treatment philosophy that encourages early dropouts to return to service if their motivation changes.
4. Using adherence contracts for high-risk clients.
5. Facilitating the client's receipt of medical care, food, housing, financial assistance, educational or vocational counseling, and job training.
6. Referring the client to case management services.
7. Conducting client satisfaction surveys.
8. Ensuring that clinical staff receive training in dealing both with substance use and psychiatric disorders.
9. Providing integrated clinical services to clients with dual disorders.

Aftercare

Aftercare helps the client maintain gains made during inpatient care, prevent relapse to substance abuse or a recurrence of psychiatric illness, or intervene early in the relapse process. Participation in aftercare is associated with better alcohol and drug use outcomes, improved psychiatric outcomes, improvement in functioning, lower relapse rates, and lower readmission rates.[18] Despite the importance of and positive outcome associated with aftercare adherence, numerous studies report serious problems in entering aftercare following completion of inpatient care.[19] Poor adherence to aftercare is common across a range of substance use disorders combined with mood disorders,[20] schizophrenia,[21] post-traumatic stress disorders,[22] and borderline and antisocial personality disorders.[23] Poor adherence contributes to clinical deterioration, which causes or exacerbates medical or psychosocial problems and contributes to the need for hospitalization.

Preparing Inpatients for Aftercare

Preparing dual diagnosis inpatients for aftercare before hospital discharge increases aftercare entry rates.[24] We found that a brief motivational therapy session provided by an outpatient clinician before hospital discharge almost doubled the initial aftercare entry rates.[25] Another group of researchers also found that a single motivational session provided to inpatients before discharge more than doubled aftercare entry rates.[26]

Rehospitalization

Although many factors impact a client's decompensation and the need for hospitalization, poor adherence with psychiatric medications and aftercare program attendance and failure to maintain abstinence from substances are frequently cited as major reasons that clients return to the hospital.[27] There is a significant subgroup of clients who are very high utilizers of treatment and are hospitalized multiple times.[28]

Chapter 7
Individual Treatment

Treatment of Psychiatric Disorders

There are many effective psychological, social, medication, and combined treatments for psychiatric disorders.[1] Treatments such as cognitive-behavioral therapy or social skills training are used with many different disorders. Other treatments are specific to a psychiatric illness, such as Personal Therapy for schizophrenia or Dialectic Behavioral Therapy for borderline personality disorder. Therapies include the following:

1. Behavioral therapy (used with many disorders).
2. Cognitive and cognitive-behavioral therapies (CBT, used with many disorders).
3. Interpersonal psychotherapy (IPT, used with many disorders).
4. Dialectical-behavioral therapy (DBT, used with borderline disorders).
5. Family and marital therapies (some are used with many disorders; some are used with a specific type of illness; some are used for marital or family problems).
6. Personal therapy (used with schizophrenia).
7. Psychiatric rehabilitation programs (used with chronic mental disorders).
8. Social rhythm therapy (used with bipolar illness, combined with IPT).
9. Social skills training (used with many disorders).
10. Supportive-expressive psychotherapy (SEP, used with many disorders).
11. Trauma-based therapies (used with PTSD or traumatic grief).

Several of these treatment approaches have incorporated interventions for psychiatric clients who have co-occurring substance use disorders. For example, Dr. Marsha Linehan, who developed DBT, wrote an additional manual for clients who have both borderline and substance use disorders. A manual on schizophrenia and addiction was added to the social skills training modules that were originally developed by Dr. Robert Liberman. Given that two-thirds of clients with borderline disorders and almost one-half with schizophrenia have a co-occurring substance use disorder, the need to adapt treatment approaches for these clients is evident.

Many clients need medications in addition to psychosocial treatments.[2] Medications are used for recurrent, chronic, and more severe acute conditions. Specific medications depend on the client's current symptoms and history of response to medicines. While some clients benefit from a single medication, others need additional medications to treat their symptoms. Recurrent and chronic conditions (e.g., schizophrenia, obsessive-compulsive disorder, bipolar illness, recurrent major depression) require maintenance medications once symptoms are in remission or well controlled.

Treatment of Substance Use Disorders

There are many effective psychosocial (individual and group therapies and "programs" involving multiple types of groups and services), medication, and combined approaches for substance use disorders. Many of these are described in therapy manuals published by the National Institute on Drug Abuse and the National Institute on Alcohol Abuse and Alcoholism.[3] These psychosocial treatments include the following:

1. Cognitive-behavioral therapy (CBT).
2. Community reinforcement approach (CRA).
3. Cue exposure (CE).
4. Group drug counseling (GDC).
5. Individual drug counseling (IDC).
6. MATRIX model (for cocaine and methamphetamine).
7. Motivational enhancement therapy (MET).
8. Motivational interviewing (MI).
9. Multi-systemic family therapy (MSFT).
10. Rational emotive therapy (RET).
11. Relapse prevention (RP).
12. Social skills training (SST, also called coping skills training).
13. Social network therapy (SNT).
14. Twelve Step facilitation therapy (TSFT).

Treatment approaches such as CBT, RET, SST, RP, and MI are used with psychiatric disorders and with substance use disorders. Most other therapies listed above were designed specifically for treating substance use disorders.

Medications are used to help the client safely and comfortably withdraw from addictive substances such as alcohol, opiates, or sedatives. Detoxification may occur in an inpatient, residential, or ambulatory setting, depending on the severity of the addiction and support system available to the client.

Medicines can be used to "replace" the addictive drug. For example, methadone maintenance (MM) helps opiate addicts transfer addiction from street drugs like heroin to methadone, which can be administered and monitored by professionals in a licensed MM clinic.[4] Nicotine replacement therapy in the form of gum (Nicorette™), patches (Nicoderm™), or nasal spray (Nicotrol™) is used with smokers to help them stop smoking.[5]

Antagonist or mixed replacement (agonist/antagonist) medications are used for opiate addicts. Naltrexone (Trexan) "antagonizes" the effects of heroin so the addict does not get high if she ingests heroin while using this drug.[6] Buprenorphine (Buprenex) has both replacement and antagonist effects.[7] This medication can be used to help the opiate addict withdraw from heroin. In addition, it can help the addict in maintenance therapy. A colleague who is a medical director of a detoxification unit recently stated that rates of heroin-addicted patients leaving detoxification against medical advice decreased significantly since using buprenorphine.

Medications may be used to reduce craving among alcoholics and those addicted to smoking. For example, naltrexone (Revia) reduces the alcoholic's craving and buproprion (Zyban) reduces the smoker's craving.[8]

For alcoholism, disulfiram (Antabuse) serves as an "aversive therapy."[9] If the alcoholic drinks with this drug in the system (it may remain in his system for up to seven to fourteen days after the last dose), he becomes sick. This aversive reaction is a motivator for some alcoholics not to drink while on this medication. By the time the medicine leaves the person's system, the desire or craving to drink may have subsided.

Medications that eliminate or reduce psychiatric symptoms such as depression or anxiety may also reduce the desire to drink or use drugs. Medications that help organize thinking can also reduce a client's desire for substances.

Clinicians can help clients in several ways vis-à-vis medications. They can encourage clients to consider using medications to aid in withdrawal, maintenance, or ongoing recovery from addiction. Clinicians can monitor and assess medication adherence in order to identify and intervene early when the client evidences poor adherence. They can also help clients anticipate and prepare for negative reactions to medications used to treat any disorder conveyed by members of mutual support groups. Finally, clinicians can collaborate with the client's physicians by reporting significant changes in symptoms or discussing strategies to improve adherence with medications.

Principles of Effective Treatment

The National Institute on Drug Abuse (NIDA) published Principles of Effective Treatment,[10] which reviews the empirically-based treatments for drug abuse and addiction and delineates principles of treatment. These principles can serve as an important guide to providing care for clients, including those with co-occurring psychiatric disorders. Following is a brief discussion of these principles:

1. *No single treatment fits all individuals.* Clients do not all respond the same to a psychosocial and/or medication treatment. Many benefit from individual and group treatment combined. Others benefit from medications and therapy.

2. *Treatment must be readily available and should address multiple needs of the client.* Easy access to treatment increases the odds that the client will adhere to the initial evaluation and early sessions. Many dual disorder clients have more problems than just a substance use disorder. These include medical, family, social, housing, economic, legal, or job problems. Case management and other services may be needed to help clients with other problems or needs.

3. *The treatment plan should be continually modified based on the changing needs and problems of the client.* Treatment is an active dynamic process. The focus may change as the client progresses through treatment or when the client has a setback or relapse.

4. *Adequate time in treatment is needed for the client to benefit.* Outcome is associated with time in treatment. Fewer than ninety days in treatment is seldom effective for drug dependent individuals. The highest risk period of drop out and relapse is the first ninety days in treatment. Using motivational and adherence strategies can help retain clients so they benefit from an adequate course of treatment.

5. *Mental disorders should be treated in an "integrated" manner.* The treatment plan needs to address both types of disorders, regardless of whether services are provided by one clinician or program. For example, if an addiction clinic does not have the capability of providing psychiatric treatment, treatment can be integrated by working closely with a mental health provider.

6. *Detoxification is only the first stage of treatment for some addicts.* This "prepares" clients for ongoing treatment. Clinicians need to facilitate entry to the next level of care, such as a rehabilitation program, halfway house, partial hospital, intensive outpatient, or outpatient program.

7. *Treatment does not have to be voluntary to be effective.* If the addicted client is in treatment, professionals have an opportunity to influence him. There is an abundance of literature showing that clients mandated to treatment by the criminal justice system benefit. Although motivation is initially external, it may shift to internal over time.

8. *Drug use should be monitored during treatment.* This provides an objective assessment of substance use. For some clients, external checking motivates them to stay sober. Progress among clients with psychiatric disorders may be hindered due to the effects of substance use. Urinalysis reports help to identify recent use and provide the clinician with "grist for the therapeutic mill."

9. *Treatment programs should assess HIV/AIDS, Hepatitis B and C, TB, and other infectious diseases.* Counseling should focus on reducing behaviors that increase the risk of transmitting or acquiring diseases (e.g., using dirty needles, cotton or rinsing water for IV users, unprotected sex, and sex with multiple partners).

10. *Recovery can be a long-term process and require multiple episodes of treatment.* Many addicted individuals remain in recovery long after completing professional treatment by attending AA, NA, DRA, or other mutual support groups. Others use multiple treatments over time as their clinical condition changes. Addicted clients are no different than those with mental disorders in that some are sicker, have more difficulty with recovery, and need more professional services than others. A client with schizophrenia or bipolar illness readmitted to the hospital as a result of symptom exacerbation faces far less judgmental and negative reactions by professionals than an addicted patient who relapses. Clinicians who lack empathy and convey negative reactions to relapsers often contribute to client's feeling guilty and shame-

ful. Therefore clinicians must work hard to convey helpful attitudes regardless of how often a client enters treatment.

Treatment of Dual Disorders

Our DDRC model integrates clinical strategies from psychiatric and addiction medicine treatment approaches. DDRC also integrates information from our clinical and quality improvement studies. In addition to our recovery oriented model for treatment, there are other models of integrated treatment. These include the following:

1. *Approaches for chronic mental illness and substance use disorders.* See Drake and colleagues, Minkoff and colleagues, Montrose and Daley, Daley and Moss, Mueser and colleagues, and Ridgely and Pepper for more detailed discussion of these models as used with chronic mental disorders.

2. *Approaches for addressing engagement, early treatment retention, and motivational issues.* See Osher and Kofoed, Daley and Zuckoff, Mueser and colleagues, and Bellack and DiClemente for discussions about how to facilitate treatment entry, improve adherence, and improve motivation among clients with dual disorders.

3. *Approaches to integrated treatment for specific types of psychiatric disorders combined with substance abuse.* For example, Ziedonis developed a model of change and model of relapse prevention for clients with schizophrenia. Najavits developed a "Seeking Safety" model for women with PTSD. Weiss developed a model for use with bipolar illness. We and our colleagues at WPIC (see Cornelius, et al; Daley, et al; Salloum, et al) developed psychosocial and combined treatment models for mood disorders and addiction. Linehan adapted her DBT model for clients with borderline personality disorders. Roberts and colleagues developed a model for use with clients with schizophrenia. All of these integrated models focus on helping clients deal with both substance use and psychiatric issues.

Length of Treatment for DDRC

In acute care and time-limited inpatient settings, most clients stay between several days and weeks. A limited number of individual sessions are available to the individual counselor. The fewer sessions available, the more focused treatment should be.

In partial hospital and outpatient settings, the length of treatment depends on the client's problems, treatment program's philosophy, and source of reimbursement. When the client first enters treatment, it is helpful to establish an initial, time-limited contract with the understanding that this contract can be reevaluated and changed as needed based on the client's progress and symptom change over time. We often use a three-month initial contract for outpatient care and four weeks for a partial hospital program. A treatment contract sets the expectation that treatment does not last indefinitely (although chronically ill clients may go in and out of treatment over a long period of time). Many counselors are use to providing long-term treatment to help clients explore important issues relevant to their disorders. However, because managed care is limiting the number of sessions a clinician can provide, shorter term contracts are being used more frequently than in the past.

Individual DDRC Session

An individual DDRC session reviews substance use and mental health recovery issues. The time spent in a given session on a specific issue varies and depends on the needs and capabilities of the client. For example, even if an anxious alcoholic client has been sober nine months, the counselor may briefly inquire about addiction recovery issues (i.e., cravings or close calls, involvement in self-help group meetings, discussions with a sponsor). If a client's anxiety has improved, the counselor may inquire about symptoms this client had before coming to treatment (anxiety, panic, depression, suicidality, energy). Any crisis issues are attended to as they emerge.

Some clients will exhibit low motivation to address the substance use disorder and prefer to focus only on their psychiatric disorder. It may take time for the counselor to develop a therapeutic relationship and be able to influence the client to also focus on substance use issues. Great patience and flexibility are needed in such cases.

The majority of the time spent in the individual counseling session focuses on the client's agenda unless a crisis takes up the session. The client is usually asked at the beginning of the session, "What concern, problem, or goal do you want to focus on in today's session?" The problem, concern, or goal should be one the client has identified in his treatment plan. The counselor helps the client explore the problem or issue to better understand and cope with it. Coping strategies are important because the session should be a purposeful one aimed at helping the client work toward self-awareness and change. During the course of the DDRC session, any "live" material that is relevant to the client's dual disorders or recovery can be processed. For example, if the client gives evidence of "maladaptive thinking" in the session contributing to anxiety or depressive symptoms such as "jumping to conclusions" or "focusing only on the negative," this can be pointed out and discussed in the context of the client's problems. If the client becomes frustrated and angry because the counselor cannot meet his unrealistic expectations or demands, the counselor can help the client understand how such attitudes and expectations affect interpersonal relationships.

The counselor can provide encouragement and feedback at the end of the session for the work that the client accomplished or for the effort put forth. Often clients have difficulty seeing progress or acknowledging their efforts at changing. Expectations are high or unrealistic, and positive changes are minimized by clients. Feedback from the counselor helps counteract this and provides the client with a more realistic view of the recovery process.

The session ends with a review of what the client will do before the next session relating to his recovery. Reading, writing, or behavioral assignments may be given at the end of the session. These therapeutic assignments get the client to actively work on problems and issues between sessions. For example, a client who has a serious problem expressing anger impulsively and inappropriately can be asked to keep a "daily anger log." This anger log is used to record situations triggering anger, the degree to which the anger is experienced, thoughts, actual actions taken, and new ideas on coping strategies. This log is reviewed during each treatment session. A client who is lonely, isolated, and depressed may be given the assigned task of initiating a social contact with one friend. A therapeutic assignment should not be too difficult or the client may feel frustrated. Assignments that have some degree of difficulty provide the best opportunity for mastery over problems.

Recovery Issues at Various Phases of Treatment

The recovery issues that follow can be reviewed in individual sessions. Specific areas of focus will depend on the client's current problems and needs, where he is in the recovery process, and the treatment contract. Short-term treatment (less than twelve sessions), for example, would be limited to just a few of these issues. Following is a brief listing of the issues associated with each phase of recovery. Although separated for purposes of discussion, there is overlap among these issues. Not all issues can be explored in treatment. Clients involved in ongoing self-help groups can continue focusing on recovery issues over time.

Phase 1—Transition and Engagement

1. Discuss symptoms and problems leading the client to treatment.
2. Help client understand the diagnoses (both psychiatric and addictive illness) and accept the reality of the dual disorders.
3. Discuss psychiatric and substance use disorders as "no fault" biopsychosocial disorders with multiple causes and effects.
4. Help client recognize an inability to consistently control the use of substances.
5. Discuss the effects of substance use on psychiatric symptoms (covering up, triggering off, or worsening psychiatric symptoms).
6. Discuss the client's thoughts and feelings about being in treatment, especially if it resulted from external pressure (family, employer, court, commitment).
7. Validate the client's ambivalence about treatment and recovery.
8. Help the client understand and accept the need for family involvement.
9. Discuss the role of medications in treatment and the client's perception of taking medications.

Phase 2—Stabilization

1. Discuss the process of stabilizing from acute psychiatric symptoms and how treatment helps short- and long-term recovery.
2. Discuss the process of getting sober and adjusting to being substance free, including what the client may miss about not using.
3. Review the benefits of sobriety.

4. Provide information on dual disorders based on the client's and family's questions or concerns.
5. Focus on acceptance of disorders and reviewing expectations of treatment.
6. Monitor and discuss cravings and "close calls" and how to manage these.
7. Monitor psychiatric symptoms and discuss strategies to manage these.
8. Discuss benefits of self-help programs and resistances; monitor attendance and participation.
9. Help the client develop a problem list.
10. Reinforce continued abstinence from substances.
11. Focus on family issues and involvement in treatment.
12. Monitor medication compliance and discuss any medication problem.

Phase 3—Early Recovery

1. Discuss strategies to deal with people, places, events, and things that represent a relapse risk for addiction.
2. Discuss strategies to manage social pressures to use substances.
3. Discuss faulty beliefs or inaccurate thinking associated with either disorder.
4. Monitor psychiatric symptoms, cravings or close calls, medication compliance, attendance and participation in self-help groups.
5. Discuss strategies to manage "persistent symptoms" of psychiatric illness.
6. Help the client identify behaviors to change and methods to change.
7. Discuss the importance of structure in daily life to keep busy, stay focused on recovery, and get involved in enjoyable leisure activities.
8. Discuss the impact of the disorders on family members and their concerns and questions.
9. Discuss grief issues and feelings of guilt and shame associated with psychiatric illness, addiction, or both.
10. Help client see progress, even in small changes.
11. Discuss any relapses or setbacks and help client learn from these.

Phase 4—Middle Recovery

1. Continue to get client to increase self-disclosure about thoughts, feelings, and problems.

2. Discuss the process of making amends to family and others hurt by behaviors.
3. Discuss other relationship problems.
4. Discuss ways to improve communication and strengthen relationships.
5. Discuss spirituality issues.
6. Continue discussing strategies to develop and/or improve cognitive and behavioral coping strategies to deal with negative or upsetting thoughts, feelings, and problems.
7. Identify warning signs of psychiatric relapse and strategies to manage these.
8. Identify warning signs of addiction lapse or relapse and strategies to manage these.
9. Continue to monitor psychiatric symptoms, cravings or close calls related to substance use, medication compliance, and participation in self-help groups.
10. Discuss strategies the client can use to monitor recovery on a daily basis.
11. Discuss any relapses or setbacks and help client learn from these.

Phase 5—Late Recovery

1. Continue to help client increase awareness of "inner self" (defenses, personality traits, values, strengths, and vulnerabilities).
2. When relevant, help client gain a greater understanding of past influences on current behaviors, values, and relationships.
3. Deal more in-depth with grief or family of origin issues.
4. Discuss the advantages of broadening support group involvement, if needed, to include ACOA or survivor groups.
5. Discuss ways to change character defects or personality traits that cause self-defeating behaviors or other problems.
6. Focus more on "lifestyle balancing" so attention is directed to all major areas of life—recovery, work, love, relationships, fun, and spirituality.

Phase 6—Maintenance

1. Discuss "giving away" what one learned in recovery by sponsoring others or serving the greater good of society.
2. Continue monitoring recovery from dual disorders and discuss problems, concerns, or setbacks.
3. Continue discussions of ways to "grow" in recovery and change oneself.
4. Discuss relapses or setbacks, and help the client learn from these.

Treatment Entry and Reengagement Strategies

Many clients do not show up for their initial assessment. Many discharged from inpatient care fail to keep their follow-up appointment for outpatient or partial hospital treatment, thus negating the gains made during hospitalization. Strategies to enhance treatment entry or reengagement and increase motivation during early recovery include:[11]

1. Using motivational interviewing or motivational enhancement therapy.
2. Using prompts to remind the client about the initial treatment session(s) (i.e., phone calls and/or letters).
3. Providing reinforcement for attending treatment sessions (i.e., bus tickets, vouchers that can be cashed in for merchandise).
4. Giving quick appointments at the time of referral.
5. Collaborating with inpatient referrals (for outpatient clinicians).
6. Helping the client deal with "other" problems (i.e., transportation, child care) that interfere with ability to attend treatment sessions.
7. Intensive contact in the early weeks of treatment (i.e., seeing the client more than once a week, providing individual and group treatment).
8. Using intensive case managers to provide outreach or help with other needs.
9. Making quick contact with clients who fail to show for appointments to offer another appointment (i.e., making phone calls or sending letters within twenty-four to forty-eight hours of the missed appointment).

Strategies for Dealing with Common Clinical Problems

Lateness is discussed with the client to determine the reasons and explore strategies for better compliance with treatment sessions. Chronic patterns of lateness can be generalized as indicative of broader problems with responsibility or as part of a self-defeating behavior.

Missed sessions are discussed to determine the reasons and to work through any resistances on the part of the client. Clients who fail to show for appointments can be called by the clinician or support staff member. A "friendly" note can be sent in the mail offering an appointment or asking the client to call. This makes it easier for the client to reengage in treatment.

Interventions with clients who come to sessions under the influence depend on their condition. Detoxification and inpatient hospitalization may be arranged in severe cases involving potential withdrawal and florid psychiatric symptoms that cannot be managed on an outpatient basis (i.e., severe mood or psychotic symptoms that interfere with the client's ability to function, suicidal attempts or plans, homicidal attempts or plans, or history of seizures or complicated withdrawal). In other cases, crisis intervention may be provided or the client may be helped to make arrangements to go home and return when sober. Limits can be set without coming across as punitive or judgmental.

Poor or noncompliance with medication (taking more or less than prescribed) is dealt with by discussing the client's reasons for not taking the medication as prescribed and the actual or potential effects on symptoms and recovery. Uncomfortable side effects or difficulty following a medication regimen, having to take multiple doses per day, or using substances are common reasons for poor compliance with medicine.

If a client does not complete a therapeutic assignment (i.e., behavioral task, reading or writing assignment), discuss the reasons and figure out whether the assigned task was too difficult. If the task was too difficult, a simpler task can be given. If the client "forgets" or has another excuse for not completing the assignment, explore this to determine the reasons. Emphasize the client's responsibility to work his recovery plan.

Some clients frequently attempt to change the focus of therapy (within or between individual treatment sessions) based on an endless number of concerns or life crises that constantly pop up. While some focus on crises is inevitable, the counselor should avoid non-focused treatment and try to keep to the structure of therapy by focusing on issues identified. This requires checking out why the client wants to change the focus of the session. A change of focus may represent avoidance or may be the client's way of saying that he is anxious about or not ready to explore a specific issue in treatment.

Treatment contracts can be used with clients around lateness, missed sessions, failure to take medications as prescribed, failure to attend medication visits, failure to complete therapeutic assignments, or coming to sessions under the influence. Clients can give their input on how these situations should be dealt with. The contract can be in writing and signed by client and clinician.

Strategies for Dealing with Denial, Resistance, or Poor Motivation

Treatment sessions can deal with ambivalence of clients regarding participation in treatment. The counselor attempts to normalize and validate ambivalence or denial in the context of addiction or psychiatric illness. Education, support, the use of therapeutic assignments, sessions with the treatment team to discuss symptoms and behaviors, and sessions involving the family or significant others may be used to help deal with denial and resistance. Any resistance is "grist for the therapeutic mill" and is explored in treatment sessions. One or several sessions of Motivational Interviewing (MI) or Motivational Enhancement Therapy (MET) can be used to enhance motivation to change.[12] MI or MET are brief approaches that can be used as "stand-alone" interventions or "added" to other interventions, usually early in the treatment process when motivation to change is more likely to be low.

Poor motivation is often a manifestation of illness, particularly with more severely addicted or psychiatrically impaired clients. Personality issues also contribute to resistance and poor motivation. The "door is left open" so clients with low motivation can reenter treatment. However limits can be set by the treatment team so the client knows that misusing treatment will not be tolerated. For example, clients who miss counseling appointments and medication visits but then call the counselor in a crisis when medications have run out may be given a physician's prescription for a week with the caveat that future refills are contingent on attending sessions with the doctor. The client is then given an appointment. Clients not seen for several months should usually not be given medication refills unless first seen by the treatment team.

Strategies for Dealing with Crises

A flexible approach is needed for dealing with crises because clients experience exacerbations of their disorders. In more severe cases, voluntary or involuntary hospitalization may be needed to stabilize a psychiatric crisis. Extra face-to-face sessions with any member of the treatment team, including the case manager for persistently mentally ill clients, may also be held. In some instances, supportive sessions via phone are held. Clients are given an emergency number that can be called 24-7 and are instructed on how and when to use the Psychiatric Emergency Room.

Substance Use Lapse and Relapse

The counselor approaches lapses or relapses as opportunities for the client to learn about relapse precipitants or set-ups. All lapses and relapses are explored to identify motivational struggles and warning signs that preceded them. Strategies are discussed to reduce relapse risk in the future. Extra sessions or phone contacts can help the client stabilize from relapse. Inpatient detoxification or rehabilitation programs may be arranged when the relapse is severe and cannot be interrupted with counseling or participation in AA, NA, or DRA.

Relapses are discussed in terms of their impact on psychiatric symptoms and recovery from dual disorders. If a client is on medication, the possible interactions with alcohol or non-prescribed drugs are discussed.

Recurrence of Psychiatric Illness

Psychiatric recurrences are reviewed in terms of warning signs and causes to help the client figure out what contributed to the symptoms. Extra sessions with the counselor or phone calls may be provided to help the client stabilize. Medication adjustments may also be made, depending on the symptoms experienced by the client.

When psychiatric symptoms are life-threatening or cause significant impairment, inpatient hospitalization is arranged. The counselor orchestrates involuntary commitment in cases where a client's welfare (or another person) is in jeopardy and the client refuses to enter voluntarily.

In any of these or similar cases, the counselor assumes a helpful, supportive, and non-judgmental stance. He also does not personalize episodes of relapse or other setbacks and accepts these as part of working with dual diagnosed clients.

Treatment Effectiveness

There is considerable evidence that treatment is effective for both psychiatric illness and addictive disorders, and "integrated" treatment is effective for dual disorders.[13] Effectiveness is defined in a variety of ways:

1. Remission of acute psychiatric symptoms.
2. Reduction of severity of chronic symptoms.
3. Cessation or reduction of substance use.
4. Reduction of high-risk behaviors putting the client at risk for transmitting or acquiring diseases or the AIDS virus.
5. Reduction of suicidal or violent behaviors.
6. Reduction of criminal or antisocial behaviors.
7. Reduction of rates of relapse or rehospitalization.
8. Improvement in treatment adherence.
9. Improvement in mental health, physical health, spiritual health, and psychosocial functioning (school, work).
10. Improvement in the quality of life.

Chapter 8
Role of the Family and Significant Others in Treatment

Effects of Dual Disorders on the Family

The family unit, individual family members, and significant others are affected by substance use, psychiatric, and dual disorders.[1] The family system is often disrupted and communication, interactions, emotional health, and financial condition of the family can be affected. With good intentions, the family may show "enabling" behaviors that help perpetuate the problems. Enabling may be "passive" when the family does nothing and accepts problematic behaviors related to the substance use or psychiatric disorder of the ill member. Or enabling may be "active" when the family covers up problems caused by this member. Sometimes this involves bailing the ill member out of legal, financial, or other trouble or assuming her responsibilities.

Dual disorders can take an emotional toll on parents, spouses, children, siblings, and other relatives. Stress can be high as a result of exposure to psychiatric symptoms or intoxicated, violent, erratic, or unpredictable behaviors. Family members may feel upset, angry, confused, anxious, worried, or depressed. Some family members, especially parents, feel guilty and responsible for causing the ill member's problems.

Children are affected by dual disorders and may have emotional, behavioral, academic, or substance abuse problems as a direct or indirect result of exposure to a parent's disorders.[2] They need education, support, and an opportunity to share some of their worries, feelings, and concerns. Children with serious problems need treatment.

Benefits of Family Involvement

Family participation is beneficial in many ways. Involving the family:

1. Allows the counselor to gather information about how family members view the disorders and their effects and how they relate to the ill member.

2. Gives the counselor an idea of the family's strengths and how it can support the ill member's recovery.

3. Provides an opportunity to figure out how the family and client get along, and how the family affects the client.

4. Provides members with an opportunity to gain information, support, and help with their own feelings and issues.

5. Helps the counselor determine if other members need an evaluation or treatment for an emotional, behavioral, or substance use problem.

Typical Concerns of Family Members

Awareness of questions and concerns of family members can aid the counselor in working with the family. These questions and concerns include the following:[3]

1. Specific diagnoses and the implications of these.
2. Causes of disorders and how substance use and psychiatric disorders interact.
3. Types of treatment and recommendations, length, excepted outcome, and cost.
4. Medications, side effects, and interactions with alcohol, street drugs, or non-prescribed drugs.
5. Family role in treatment in supporting the ill member's recovery.
6. Family member's role in treatment for their own needs, problems, and concerns.
7. How to deal with violence or the threat of it, suicidal action or the threat of it, or more severe symptoms of the disorders.
8. Whether other family members are vulnerable to psychiatric illness, substance abuse, or both, especially offspring.
9. Whether the ill family member will be able to function at a job, school, or home.
10. How to deal with emotional reactions toward the dual disorder family member (i.e., anger, disappointment, worry).
11. How to deal with the ill member who refuses help or fails to comply with treatment.
12. How to deal with psychiatric relapse.
13. How to deal with alcohol or drug relapse.
14. When detoxification or psychiatric hospitalization are needed.

Types of Family Treatment

There are a variety of family treatments that can be used, depending on the client's situation and the availability of services in a program. These include the following: [4]

1. Psychoeducational (PE) programs that provide information on dual disorders and recovery, and ways the family can cope with its concerns regarding the ill family member. These are offered to several families and can be held regularly, such as once a week or on a periodic basis such as monthly or bi-monthly. PE programs can last a half day or a full day.
2. Family therapy where issues and problems within a specific family are explored from a family systems perspective.
3. Couples therapy or parent-child therapy where specific problems between a dyad are explored.

4. Multiple family groups that combine psychoeducation, support, and discussion of mutual problems and concerns of families.

5. Exposure to family support groups for addiction such as Al-Anon, Naranon, Alateen, Alatots, Parents groups, or Codependency Anonymous.

6. Exposure to family support groups for mental illness such as NAMI (National Alliance of the Mentally Ill) groups.

Some clients are disengaged from their families and have no one whom they can involve in treatment. Families may refuse to get involved in treatment, especially those who feel tired or burned out. Family members with serious illnesses themselves (psychiatric or substance use disorders) may be unable or refuse to engage in treatment.

Family resistance to treatment or client resistance to family involvement in treatment should not be taken at face value. There are effective strategies to engage the family in treatment. Patience, persistence, and creativity are often needed on the part of the clinician.

Principles and Strategies for Helping Families

A professional does not have to be a social worker or family therapist to help a family. The following principles and strategies may help guide clinicians in working with families.

1. Do not label the family as "sick, dysfunctional, or codependent." View them as allies in the treatment process.

2. Establish contact with the family as early as possible in the assessment and treatment processes.

3. View the engagement process as important. If a family cannot be engaged in treatment, the best treatment available will not benefit them.

4. Be patient and flexible with families. Use outreach phone calls and ask families for help in working with the client. Do not rely on the client to invite the family to sessions, as the client may sabotage the chances of the family showing up.

5. Be accessible to families. Offer evening appointments, if convenient. Family groups can be held on weekends. Be available by phone as needed.

6. Focus on family strengths. Do not emphasize family deficits or problems at the expense of overlooking their strengths.

7. Provide a framework for the family to understand what is happening to the client and family system. Educating the family about substance use and psychiatric disorders, the course of illness, and recovery is an excellent way to provide this framework. Use the no-fault, biopsychosocial model of illness.

8. Connect emotionally with family members by letting them know you understand their feelings, concerns, and worries. Give them an opportunity to express their feelings. This will make it easier to help explore how to cope with feelings and adapt to the ill member's recovery.

9. Provide hope by discussing how treatment benefits clients and their families.

10. Provide a realistic view on treatment and recovery. Prepare the family for the possibility of setbacks and relapses. If relevant, discuss issues around involuntary commitment in cases when the ill member is at risk for suicide or homicide or if functioning has decompensated severely and the client is unable to take care of basic needs.

11. Link the family with family support groups in the community.

12. Link the family with other resources in the community (i.e., social services agencies, housing agencies).

13. If the client has children, educate the family members on the impact of dual disorders on their kids. Encourage the parents to talk with their children about the disorders and how they have experienced these. Parents can elicit thoughts, feelings, and questions from their kids. If a child is abusing substances or appears to have a serious mental health problem, help the parents arrange for an evaluation of this child.

Chapter 9
Overview of Group Treatments

Goals of Group Treatment

There are a variety of group treatments for psychiatric substance use and dual disorders.[1] Groups help clients explore common problems and concerns, and learn skills to manage their disorders. Issues or problems discussed in groups can also be explored in individual sessions.

Groups should provide a balance on the psychiatric and substance use disorders. However, a specific group session may focus mainly on one of these disorders. The interrelationship between the disorders is emphasized when appropriate.

Although each type of group has a particular format and objectives, the goals of group treatments may involve any of the following:

1. *Education:* provide information on psychiatric illness, alcohol and drugs, substance use disorders, treatment, and recovery from dual disorders.

2. *Self-awareness:* increase the client's self-awareness so he can relate to the material in a personal way and become aware of issues or problems that he needs to address.

3. *Motivation:* help the client understand how motivation impacts on recovery, develop motivation to change, and accept the need for treatment and self-help programs (i.e., AA, NA, DRA, or mental health support groups).

4. *Change:* facilitate change in the client's attitudes, behaviors, and coping skills.

5. *Skill development:* help the client develop or improve cognitive, emotional, behavioral, and life skills.

The amount of focus on each of these areas depends on the type of group treatment. For example, open-ended process or psychotherapy groups focus on self-awareness and problem-solving strategies while psychoeducational and skill groups focus on providing information and helping the client learn recovery skills, such as how to refuse pressures to use substances, manage anxiety, cope with boredom, or improve relationships.

Types and Structure of Dual Recovery Groups

Groups for treating dual disorders include process or psychotherapy groups, creative and expressive therapy groups, coping skills and psychoeducational groups, stress management, client-led groups, family groups, and self-help groups. Therapy groups are less structured than psychoeducational groups.

Both the content and process are important components of group. Content refers to the "what" of group, i.e., the topics, issues, problems, or skills reviewed in the group treatment sessions. Process refers to the "how" of group, i.e., the way the group is conducted and how the clients interact. Open discussion of problems of clients, lectures, behavioral role plays, monodramas, review of workbook and written assignments, and the use of creative media are ways to explore problems or issues in treatment groups. Group process issues such as members' avoidance of emotionally charged issues or how group members interact can also be discussed.

Dual recovery groups are interactive and engage clients in the group process by sharing their experiences, problems, and feelings and learning coping skills. It is therapeutic for clients to share and explore their problems and concerns, trust others, or lean on them.

Therapeutic assignments may be given during or between group sessions. These include bibliotherapy, journals or logs, workbooks, or other assignments.

Groups can be conducted with one or two leaders. Coleading groups is an excellent way of helping staff members learn to improve their skills.

The types of group programming provided depend on the treatment setting and time available. Programs in acute care hospitals are short-term, lasting less than two weeks. Partial hospital programs usually last two to six weeks. Outpatient programs are more variable. The longer time counselors have clients in treatment, the more extensive group programming can be provided.

Following is a brief description of group treatments. These groups can be adapted to inpatient, partial hospital, intensive outpatient, or outpatient settings. Groups can be adapted for various levels of functioning. For example, lower functioning clients can benefit from a group that is concrete and limited in the focus. Clients will feel more comfortable and able to participate than they would in a group with higher functioning clients who are more verbal and insightful.

Psychotherapy Groups

Psychotherapy group, also referred to as "process group," is an unstructured group that provides clients with an opportunity to discuss their problems, concerns, and feelings. Clients take responsibility to identify problems or recovery issues to work on. Varieties of intrapersonal and interpersonal issues are addressed in these groups. These groups can be conducted with men and women together. Or gender specific groups can be provided.

In addition to the problems or issues raised by clients, "process" issues can be discussed as they emerge during the course of the group session. Examples include a group member's passivity, tendency to dominate or not listen to others, conflicts between group members, or other interpersonal behaviors observed in the group by the leader.

In inpatient, partial hospital, or intensive outpatient programs, this group is usually offered at least once each program day week for an hour to an hour and a half. In outpatient treatment, this group is usually held once a week for an hour and a half. A variation for an outpatient group is to use half the session time to review a psychoeducational topic and half for open discussion of members' problems or concerns.

Creative and Expressive Therapy Groups

These groups explore problems and issues through the use of music, writing, drawing, painting, or clay. Group sessions can be unstructured and open-ended or can be structured on a specific theme or recovery issue (i.e., cravings, relapse, support systems, feelings). Such groups are often a "safe" way for clients to identify and express personal issues. Creative media helps clients tap unconscious material. Finished products and client participation in the group process provides counselors with a wealth of information about clients.

Milieu Groups

These groups are used in inpatient or residential settings. They can be led by staff or clients. We have used the following milieu groups in our programs.

1. *A morning community focus group* reviews the rules of the program, the treatment activities for the day, assigns tasks to members of the community, and provides members with the opportunity to state a goal they wish to work on during the day. Clients can complete a written daily goal planning worksheet to help guide them through this process. New members can be introduced and those being discharged can say their good-byes and review their follow-up plans. This group can be held up to seven days a week in inpatient or residential settings.

2. *An evening community focus group* reviews the day in treatment. Each client comments on the goal set at the beginning of the day. Community concerns are also discussed in this meeting. Clients can share positive feedback, words of encouragement, or thank others for positive things they have done during the day. This group can be held up to seven days a week.

3. *A community group* is one in which clients and staff members discuss issues pertinent to the entire treatment community. If there are client-elected officers in the milieu, they assume responsibility for running the meeting and ensure that client concerns are brought up for discussion with staff. Staff can bring up issues that affect the milieu and reinforce program rules, policies, and philosophy. Regular community meetings may help prevent little issues from becoming big ones that could have an adverse impact on the community. Community groups can be held weekly or when there are serious problems on the unit that are disruptive to the overall community.

Relapse Prevention or Skill Groups

Relapse prevention and skill groups can be used throughout the continuum of care. Many of these overlap with the psychoeducational groups discussed in the next section.

1. *Coping with feelings* groups review cognitive and behavioral strategies to help clients manage feelings such as anxiety, guilt and shame, depression, boredom, and anger. Multiple sessions can be offered on each of these feelings to ensure sufficient time is

spent on emotional management strategies. Clients show the greatest interest in the sessions on anxiety, depression, and anger.

2. *Relapse prevention* groups teach clients to anticipate and cope with the possibility of psychiatric or substance relapse. Group sessions may be provided on any of the following topics: understanding and managing relapse warning signs, understanding and managing high-risk relapse factors, craving and impulse control, coping with negative thinking, refusing alcohol and drug use offers, developing a recovery network, leisure planning, and developing an aftercare plan. Coping with alcohol or drug lapse or relapse or psychiatric relapse are also discussed.

3. *Cognitive therapy* groups review methods to change cognitive distortions or inaccurate thinking that contribute to depression, anxiety, substance abuse, or other problems. Problems in thinking presented by clients are used to teach cognitive methods.

4. *Problem-solving* groups teach clients a problem-solving process that can be applied to different life problems. Specific problems presented by clients are used to teach this method.

5. *Stress management* groups review strategies to manage stress without using alcohol or other drugs.

Psychoeducational Groups

Psychoeducational (PE) group sessions can be used in inpatient, residential, partial hospital, or outpatient settings. A specific PE group treatment curriculum can be developed for use in any treatment setting (see the next chapter for specific PE group curriculum on 43 group topics). PE group programs can vary in terms of number of sessions offered per week and total number of sessions offered during the treatment course. For example, clients in our various inpatient or residential dual disorders programs participate in five to fifteen PE groups a week.

PE groups provide information on recovery and help clients explore coping strategies to manage the issues reviewed in groups. It is important to balance the focus on "problems" and "coping strategies" so clients are exposed to practical strategies that help them deal with their problems. Each PE session has a recovery topic with objectives and key points to cover. Recovery workbook assignments are used so clients relate to the topic in a personal way.

Self-Help Groups

Clients should be provided information on self-help groups for addiction (AA, NA, CA, Women for Sobriety, Rational Recovery), dual diagnosis (Double Trouble, Dual Recovery Anonymous, SAMI, CAMI, MISA), and mental health disorders (Emotions Anonymous, Recovery Inc., and support groups for specific types of illness such as anxiety, mood, or schizophrenic disorders). Clients should also be exposed to support groups meetings within the treatment setting if available and in the community. If possible, visits to local "recovery clubs" are recommended.

Family Groups

A multiple family group (MFG) provides several families information about dual disorders and recovery, an opportunity to discuss concerns and problems and offer support to one another. This group can be offered in any treatment setting on a weekly, biweekly, or monthly basis. An MFG can be structured around a specific theme or topic related to dual disorders and recovery but should also offer a chance for participants to discuss issues important to them. MFG sessions should be held at a time convenient to families and can last up to two hours. They usually include clients although some MFG sessions have been solely for family members.

Another type of MFG is a family psychoeducational workshop (FPW). This is similar to an MFG in terms of the aims. The main difference is that a FPW can last much longer, up to an entire day. This provides staff with an opportunity to cover a wide range of topics while allowing plenty of time for the sharing of issues and support among the various families. Workshops can be offered monthly or on a variable basis, depending on the needs of the families.

Recreational Groups

Recreational groups help clients learn to have fun without alcohol or drugs. They keep them busy too. These groups offer a chance for clients to practice social skills. This is helpful for shy, isolated, or withdrawn clients who keep to themselves. Although counselors can offer specific types of recreational activities for clients to engage in, getting them to plan and carry out activities themselves has a greater impact.

Problems Frequently Discussed in DDRC Group Sessions

A list of the common problems brought up in group treatment sessions is presented below.[2] Counselors can include "open-discussion" time for these problems as part of a structured psychoeducational group program, particularly if group sessions are for one and one half hours or longer. One approach is to use half the group time to cover the curriculum or topic and use the other half for discussion of problems raised by group members. Psychotherapy groups are designed so that participants identify personal problems and issues to explore during group time.

1. *Motivational struggles.* These include lowered desire for recovery or difficulty making changes. Motivational problems show in denial or minimization of either disorder, poor adherence with treatment sessions or self-help group attendance, and failure to accept abstinence as the goal. Poor adherence contributes to substance use or psychiatric relapse.

2. *Strong desires, obsessions, or craving to use substances.* These are more common in the beginning stages of recovery although clients with months or longer of recovery can experience strong desires to use substances.

3. *Lapse or relapse to alcohol or other drug use.* It is not uncommon for group members to lapse or relapse, especially during the early months of recovery. It takes time to develop motivation and coping skills needed to reduce relapse risk.

4. *Psychiatric relapse.* Symptoms may return or worsen despite involvement in treatment. Many factors, including substance use, can impact relapse. Poor compliance with medications and therapy are factors contributing to recurrence of psychiatric illness.

5. *Frustration with treatment or a slow response.* Clients sometimes feel their progress is too slow or that treatment is ineffective. Sometimes, problems in a relationship with a professional caregiver (i.e., counselor or psychiatrist) are discussed.

6. *Problems related to self-help participation.* Members vary in their participation in self-help programs. While attendance is encouraged, active participation enables clients to gain the maximum from these programs. Some clients refuse to attend, attend only occasionally, or participate minimally. Group members may discuss conflicts with a sponsor or members of a self-help program.

7. *Relationship problems.* Interpersonal problems with family, friends, or colleagues are frequently the topic of group discussion. These problems run the gamut from mildly distressing to severe. Some of these problems pose a threat to recovery or well-being. Examples include interpersonal conflicts, anger or disappointment at others, emotional or physical violence, inappropriate sexual interactions (i.e., unprotected sex, sex with a stranger, promiscuity), involvement in relationships that are non-supportive or characterized by lack of reciprocity, difficulty saying no or setting limits with others, and difficulty asking others for help or support.

8. *Upsetting emotional states. Problems with mood states or feelings are common among many clients.* Many group members are not accustomed to managing distress or handling feelings while being substance free. The inability to manage emotions effectively accounts for the greatest percentage of relapses to substance use following a period of recovery. Group members benefit from learning emotional management skills, such as identifying, recognizing and accepting feelings, and learning to live with them without using substances. With chronic and recurrent psychiatric disorders, some mood symptoms may never remit totally, which requires the client to manage persistent symptoms, such as anxiety or depression.

9. *Boredom with recovery.* Some clients become easily bored with recovery. They feel life is not better despite being sober.

10. *Other psychosocial problems.* These include problems related to school, work, housing, finances, the legal system, or how to structure leisure time.

Managing Problems in the Group Process

The counselor may encounter problems in the process of conducting treatment groups that need addressed for the group to function effectively. Following is a review of common problems in groups and strategies to handle these.

1. *A group focuses only on substance use problems.* The counselor must make sure that group sessions are reasonably balanced, and focus on both psychiatric and substance related problems. This does not imply a fifty-fifty balance, as more or less

attention may be paid to substance use or psychiatric disorders at various points in time. If the counselor feels the group is too focused on the substance use problems, she can ask group members to discuss how substance-related issues affect their psychiatric disorder or recovery.

2. *A group focuses only on psychiatric problems or symptoms.* The same strategy discussed above can be used in situations where the group avoids addressing substance use issues. The counselor can ask group members how psychiatric symptoms affect the desire to use substances or how these symptoms affect the recovery process.

3. *A member dominates group discussion or brings the discussion back to himself.* The counselor can thank the member for the contributions and then elicit opinions and experiences from other group members. If the group member persistently tries to dominate group discussions or always turns the discussion back to his own problems or issues, this behavior pattern can be pointed out by the counselor to make this member and other group members aware of the behavior. Other members can be asked how they feel about the member dominating the discussion and how they want to deal with this in a way that is satisfying to everyone in the group. Although this creates a problem, some group members find that it creates a safety net for them because they believe they do not have to self-disclose personal problems or feelings as long as another member is taking up group time.

4. *A member does not disclose any problem or open up in the group session.* The counselor can share his observations about this member's behavior, generalize the issues by group members to talk about difficulties with self-disclosing (i.e., shame, shyness, social anxiety). Discussion can then focus on ways that group members who have trouble self-disclosing can gradually learn to trust the group and self-disclose their personal thoughts, feelings, problems, or concerns.

5. *A member rejects the input, advice, or feedback of other group members.* The counselor can point out this pattern and engage the group in a discussion of why this pattern is occurring and implications of it. Members who offer help and support only to have their attempts rejected can be asked to talk about what this feels like so the member rejecting their help is aware of the impact of this behavior on others.

6. *A member only pays attention when the discussion focuses on his problems or interrupts others when they talk.* The counselor can point out his observations of the group member and discuss the reasons for this behavior. The group can then engage in a discussion of the effects of this behavior (i.e., upsets other members, turns them off, makes them feel like their problems are not important) and the importance of "giving and receiving" mutual support by listening to one another's concerns and problems.

7. *A member wants easy answers to problems or is quick to provide easy solutions to others when they discuss personal problems.* The counselor can share his observations of these patterns and ask the group to discuss the importance of taking responsibility to find solutions to their problems and to identify more than one strategy

to address a particular problem. The leader can emphasize that while there are many different alternative ways to resolve specific problems, seldom are there easy or simple solutions, and that time, patience, and persistence are needed for group members to adequately resolve problems. When a group member provides an easy solution, the group counselor can acknowledge this is one strategy that may help some people, but it is also helpful to have other strategies. The counselor can then engage the group in a discussion of other strategies to resolve the problem under discussion. Finally, the group counselor can emphasize to the group that learning a problem-solving process is as important as dealing with specific problems because everyone will face problems in recovery.

8. *A group member believes that individual treatment and/or medications are the main form of treatment.* It is not unusual for some clients to devalue group sessions and prefer individual treatment. Some believe that medications are the answer, that any change in symptoms or feelings can be addressed by changing the medication dosage or adding another medication. The counselor can acknowledge the group member's position and reiterate that a comprehensive approach to treatment involves a variety of interventions, including group sessions. The member can be encouraged to try a half dozen or more group sessions to give these sessions a chance to help. The counselor can also elicit experiences of other group members, especially those the counselor knows have benefited from group sessions.

9. *A member tries to use the group counselor for individual therapy during the group session.* The counselor can ask other group members to comment on the problems or issues presented by this member to engage the group in the discussion. Group members can also be asked how they relate to the problem or issue presented on a personal level. If the group member asks the counselor how to handle a specific problem, he can encourage the member to directly ask peers in the group their ideas on dealing with this problem.

10. *Members arrive late for the group session or want to leave during discussions.* The leader and group should decide on a rule regarding lateness to group. Sometimes, there are legitimate reasons for being late (i.e., the bus a member takes was running fifteen minutes late, the member had a flat tire). Members may be given a break once or twice for being late. Or the group may establish a rule where the member cannot join the group after a certain amount of time (i.e., more than ten minutes after the start of the group). If time limits are not set, some members may consistently be late. Members who are persistently late can be asked to discuss this pattern of behavior, how it shows in other areas of life, and what they think needs to be done to change this pattern. Group members should not leave the session unless a true emergency occurs (i.e., they have a minor illness and need to use the restroom). Routinely allowing people to walk in and out disrupts the flow of the conversation and gives the message that what members say is not important. Members leave group sessions due to boredom, feeling like the discussions do not relate to them, or to avoid focusing on their personal issues or problems.

11. *The group talks in generalities and avoids exploring specific problems in-depth.* The counselor can point out this dynamic to the group members and ask them to

discuss why they are not talking about specific problems or concerns. Members can then be asked to set the agenda by identifying specific problems or concerns for group discussion. Group members may view counseling groups as no different than open discussions in self-help meetings.

12. *The group avoids confronting a member who behaves inappropriately.* The counselor can point out this dynamic and ask the group members what they think about the inappropriate behavior and what led to their avoiding it.

Other problems may occur during group time, but these are the ones we have observed the most frequently over years of reviewing hundreds of group sessions. We wish to stress again that while the "content" (i.e., problems and issues discussed) of the group is important, if the "process" bogs down, not much will get accomplished. Some group members may miss sessions or drop out as a result. Because group members may avoid these issues directly, the group counselor will not always know the reasons for a member's poor attendance or early drop out from group. In our experience, it is not uncommon for members to be upset over process issues. A "preventive" strategy is to periodically engage the group in a discussion about the group process. The group counselor can ask members what they think about the group sessions, what they like and dislike about how the group has been going, and what they would like to see different in how the group members work together.

Team Communication

Group leaders and individual counselors should regularly communicate to share information regarding clients. This can be done during team meetings, by phone, informally at the program site as staff members encounter one another, or through brief written notes. For example, one clinician who conducts groups that other clinicians' clients attend uses a brief checklist that states the client's name; whether or not the client attended, canceled, or failed to show for group; and any clinically significant information (i.e., client expresses an increase in suicidal ideation or reports a relapse to alcohol or drug use).

Developing a Dual Diagnosis Group Program

A dual diagnosis program involving a variety of groups is an excellent way to provide comprehensive services to clients and families.[3] A group program should be based on the diagnoses, problems, and level of functioning of clients; staff interest and availability; and length of stay of clients in treatment.

Staff from all disciplines should be involved in developing and conducting group programming. Even if a few select staff members are designated as "primary" group leaders, others can be involved. For example, a psychiatrist or psychologist can provide a group on causes and treatments of psychiatric illness, a physician's assistant or nurse can provide a group on medical aspects of alcohol and other drugs, or a social worker can provide a group on the impact of dual disorders on the family. Ancillary staff can contribute to a group program. For example, a pharmacist can provide a group on medication education or a group on the effects of alcohol and drugs on psychiatric medications. Or a priest, minister, or rabbi can provide a group on spirituality.

Some staff will be resistant to conducting groups because they feel inadequate, lack training in group treatments, do not value groups, or feel they are too busy and do not have the time to conduct group sessions. Strategies for working through this resistance include getting staff members to participate in the planning of the group program, offering them education and training, providing an experienced group coleader, setting the expectation that conducting group treatments is part of the job description, and providing regular group supervision. Over time, many staff members will be able to work through their resistance.

Clients will sometimes be resistant to group treatments. In most cases, this resistance can be dealt with by providing an orientation about group treatments, discussing how groups can aid recovery, and discussing concerns and fears of a client regarding group participation. Occasionally, a client may evidence extreme anxiety and fear of talking in groups and may have to be held out of groups until this anxiety is under control. In inpatient settings clients who are psychotic or manic need to stabilize before attending group sessions.

Some groups can be based on the level of functioning or time that clients have been sober. For example, in one of our programs, lower functioning clients attend a separate dual recovery group than higher functioning clients. In another program, an advanced recovery group is offered to clients with several months of sobriety. This provides them an opportunity to focus on issues that would be difficult to address in a group whose members have been unable to establish sobriety. We offer stabilization and clean-start groups to clients entering outpatient treatment. These focus on practical issues pertinent to stabilizing from psychiatric symptoms and achieving abstinence.

The group program can be modified over time as staff members learn what works and what does not work with their client population. Eliciting client and family input is helpful in assessing their satisfaction with current group programming.

An orientation guide describing group treatments provides clients with information about types of groups, how they work, and how they can benefit the client. This information can decrease some of their fears about groups.

It is important for clients to have access to individual treatment in addition to groups. Clients feel cheated if individual sessions are not regularly provided. Although many do well in groups, they often have problems or issues that are easier to self-disclose in an individual session. One of the authors (DD) has talked with more than a thousand clients in small focus groups in inpatient, partial hospital, and outpatient programs to ask about their experiences in treatment and find out what they would like to see different. The most common criticism expressed is inadequate time in individual counseling sessions. While some programs offer individual sessions in addition to group, many rely solely on group. A combined approach is recommended. This does not mean clients receive an equal number of individual and group sessions. It may mean, for example, that a client who attends weekly outpatient group for three months is offered three to six individual sessions. Or a client in a residential or partial program may be offered several individual sessions per week.

Chapter 10
Dual Recovery Psychoeducational Group Topics

Psychoeducational (PE) group sessions are structured around a specific recovery issue or theme related to psychiatric, substance use, or dual disorders. The specific themes reviewed depend on the total sessions available for the client. Each PE group is structured as follows:

1. Topic or recovery theme.
2. Objectives or purpose of PE group session.
3. Major points to review during the PE group session.
4. Recovery workbook assignments that are read aloud, completed, and/or discussed in group, allowing members to relate personally to the group topic, or assignments may be given to clients to complete following the group session.

The group leader reviews the material in an interactive way so that clients ask questions, share personal experiences, and provide help and support to one another. Outpatient and partial hospital PE groups last one to one and one-half hours; inpatient PE group sessions last one hour.

Before reviewing the PE group topic material in outpatient groups, the leader first takes time to discuss whether or not any clients have had setbacks, lapses or relapses, close calls, strong cravings to use substances, or any other pressing issues since the last session. Some time is spent discussing these before reviewing the group curriculum. However, since this is not a therapy group, the leader should make sure that ample time is left for covering the PE group curriculum.

Following are examples of topics or recovery themes that can be explored in PE group sessions. Each session has a curriculum that follows this section of the manual. Most of these topics have specific sections in the client guide written by one of the authors (DD) titled *Dual Diagnosis Workbook: Recovery Strategies for Substance Use and Mental Health Disorders*, (available from Independence Press, 1-800-767-8181 or *www.drdenniscdaley.com*). Specific group topics can be covered in more than one session if needed. For example, anger, anxiety, depression, and relapse are issues often requiring several sessions. If the group leader has a limited number of sessions available, he should choose topics most relevant to the client population served.

Following is a list of group topics discussed in this treatment manual.

1. Overview of Dual Disorders
2. Understanding Psychiatric Illness
3. Understanding Addiction
4. Effects of Dual Disorders
5. Medical Effects of Alcohol and Drugs
6. Withdrawal from Alcohol and Other Drugs
7. Alcohol and Other Depressants
8. Cocaine and Other Stimulants
9. Heroin and Other Opiates

10. Psychosocial Effects of Alcohol and Drugs
11. How to Use Treatment: Keys to Successful Recovery
12. Phases of Recovery
13. Developing a Problem List
14. Setting Treatment Goals
15. Advantages of Recovery
16. Denial in Addiction and Psychiatric Illness
17. Roadblocks in Recovery
18. Recovery from Dual Disorders
19. Managing Cravings for Alcohol or Drugs
20. Managing People, Places, Events, and Things
21. Managing Persistent Psychiatric Symptoms
22. Managing Anger
23. Managing Anxiety and Worry
24. Managing Boredom
25. Managing Depression
26. Managing Guilt and Shame
27. Sharing Positive Feelings in Recovery
28. Dual Disorders and the Family
29. Impact of Disorders on Children
30. Impact of Dual Disorders on Relationships
31. Saying No to Getting High
32. Resisting Pressures to Stop Taking Psychiatric Medications
33. Building a Recovery Network
34. Self-Help Programs
35. Changing Negative or Inaccurate Thinking
36. Changing Self-Defeating Behaviors
37. Changing Personality Problems
38. Developing Spirituality
39. Using a Daily Plan in Recovery
40. Financial Issues in Dual Recovery
41. Managing Relapse Warning Signs
42. Managing High Risk Relapse Factors
43. Coping with Emergencies and Setbacks

Group leaders can develop and add new group ideas as needed, based on the needs and concerns of their clients. Any of the above themes may be explored in individual DDRC sessions. These topics can also be reviewed in weekly or biweekly multiple family groups or PE workshops (half day or full day) attended by clients and families or significant others.

Psychoeducational groups can integrate reading and workbook assignments and educational videos when possible. Using a multimedia approach helps educate clients and review coping skills necessary for sober living and management of psychiatric illness.

An interactive approach is recommended to actively engage clients in discussions of recovery issues and coping strategies. Interactive methods include the following:

1. Asking clients to share their personal experiences related to the topic under discussion (e.g., depression, relapse, family, relationships).

2. Asking clients to identify coping strategies for problems discussed.
3. Engaging clients in behavioral role plays (i.e., to resist social pressure to use drugs, express positive feelings, or ask questions of the doctor).
4. Getting clients to identify cognitive distortions and practice challenging these (i.e., making mountains out of molehills).
5. Asking clients to share specific answers to workbook assignments.

An interactive approach keeps clients interested in the discussion. And, it requires them to take the responsibility to relate to material presented and discussed. At the end of each PE group session are recommendations for recovery workbook, readings, and educational videos that can be used to teach the content of the specific group topic.

PE Group Topic #1
Overview of Dual Disorders

Objectives

1. Define "dual" or "co-occurring" disorders and review their prevalence.
2. Identify types and causes of substance use disorders.
3. Identify types and causes of psychiatric disorders.
4. Identify relationships between substance use and psychiatric disorders.
5. Review treatment approaches for dual disorders.

Points for Discussion

1. Define dual or co-occurring disorders as a combination of a substance use disorder (SUD) and psychiatric (mental) disorder.
2. Review prevalence data for SUDs and co-occurring psychiatric illness.
    - Over 16 percent of adults will experience an SUD at some point in their lives. Alcohol abuse and dependence are the most common SUDs.
    - Fifty-three percent of people with a drug use disorder and 37 percent of people with an alcohol use disorder will have a psychiatric disorder during their lifetime.
    - Many have three to five disorders, hence the term "co-occurring."
3. Types of substance use disorders include:
    - Substance intoxication or withdrawal.
    - Substance abuse.
    - Substance dependence (sometimes called addiction).
    - Substance induced mental disorders (depression, psychosis).
4. Ask clients for examples of symptoms of SUDs such as withdrawal, tolerance changes, obsession, compulsion, cravings, loss of control, inability to stop, and continued use despite medical or psychosocial problems.
5. Review prevalence data for psychiatric illness.
    - More than 22 percent of adults experience a psychiatric disorder during their lifetime. Many clients have more than one psychiatric disorder. Depression and anxiety disorders are the most common.
    - There are high rates of co-occurring SUDs among clients with psychiatric illness. The highest rates are with personality disorders, bipolar illness, and schizophrenia.

6. Each psychiatric disorder has a cluster of symptoms relating to thinking, mood, behavior, and/or ability to function. Review the following DSM categories:
   - *Mood disorders*: depression, mania, and mixed states. About one-third of people with depression and 60 percent of people with mania have an SUD during their lifetime.
   - *Anxiety disorders*: generalized anxiety, phobias, panic disorder, obsessive–compulsive disorder, and posttraumatic stress disorder. Up to one-third or more of those with an anxiety disorder have an SUD during their lifetime.
   - *Psychotic disorders*: schizophrenia, schizoaffective disorder, and other psychotic disorders. Almost one-half of those with schizophrenia have an SUD during their lifetime.
   - *Personality disorders*: antisocial, borderline, narcissistic, histrionic, paranoid, schizoid, avoidant, dependent, obsessive–compulsive, and "mixed." About 85 percent of those with an antisocial and more than 65 percent with a borderline disorder have an SUD.
   - *Other psychiatric disorders*: eating disorders, compulsive gambling, impulse control, attention deficit, and adjustment disorders.
7. *Biological, psychological, and social factors* contribute to the development and maintenance of psychiatric and SUDs.
8. *Biological and physical factors* include hereditary predisposition, brain chemistry, and medical conditions.
   - First-degree relatives of those with a psychiatric or SUD have increased odds of having one of these disorders.
   - In the case of psychiatric illness, there may be disturbances in the way neurotransmitters work in the brain or excesses or deficits of these brain chemicals.
   - Medical conditions such as cancer, diabetes, or chronic pain can also contribute to psychiatric disorders.
   - In the case of addiction, drugs can "hijack" the reward center of the brain making substance use more pleasurable than eating, sex, or social activities. Cravings for substances can be intense and cause the addicted person to repeat the behavior of ingesting alcohol or drugs.
9. *Psychological factors* include defense mechanisms, personality, sensitivity to stress or how a person manages stress, and a person's beliefs and cognitive style (e.g., how a person views himself, the world, and his problems).
10. *Social factors and life experiences* impact on psychiatric illness. These include:
    - The influence of the family, other people, and the culture.
    - Losses (e.g., relationships, jobs, financial stability) and life experiences.
    - Exposure to a single trauma (e.g., rape, assault, natural disaster, or serious accident) or repeated traumatic experiences (e.g., violence, childhood abuse, sexual abuse, combat) can contribute to psychiatric illness.

11. Ask clients how their psychiatric disorders affected their substance use and how their substance use affected their psychiatric symptoms.

12. Discuss the relationships between these disorders.
    - Each illness raises the risk of developing the other.
    - Each illness affects recovery from the other.
    - Chronic alcohol or drug use can cause or worsen psychiatric symptoms, mask them, or cause a psychiatric relapse.
    - Each illness can become closely linked with the other over time.
    - Each illness can develop at separate points in time.

13. *Option*: have group members discuss previous treatment experiences when only one of their disorders was addressed. Use this to emphasize the importance of addressing both disorders in recovery.

14. Discuss approaches to treatment of dual disorders.
    - Parallel: client receives mental health treatment and substance abuse treatment in different agencies.
    - Sequential: client gets one disorder treated, then the other.
    - Integrated: both disorders are treated by the same team in the same treatment setting. This is usually the recommended approach, although other approaches may be used at different times.

15. A continuum of care is needed to treat dual disorders. This continuum includes inpatient psychiatric, inpatient detoxification, short- and long-term residential, partial hospital, intensive outpatient, and outpatient treatment. Medications and electroshock therapy are helpful treatments for many clients. Other services such as vocational rehabilitation or case management are often needed. Self-help groups (Recovery, Inc.; Emotions Anonymous; or groups for a specific type of illness) are valuable resources that aid recovery.

Supporting Materials

Dennis C. Daley and F. Campbell, *Coping with Dual Disorders*, 2nd ed. Center City, Minnesota: Hazelden. 1-800-328-9000.

Dennis C. Daley and Michael E. Thase, *Dual Disorders Recovery Workbook*. pp. 10–16. Independence, Missouri: Herald House/Independence Press, 2000. 1-800-767-8181.

PE Group Topic #2
Understanding Psychiatric Illness

Objectives

1. Define and identify types of mental or psychiatric illness.
2. Review major symptoms associated with various types of illness.
3. Identify factors contributing to psychiatric illness.
4. Review treatments for psychiatric illness.

Points for Discussion

1. Discuss psychiatric illness as a mental disorder or mental disease that involves mood, cognitive, physical, or behavioral symptoms.
2. About 22.4 percent of adults in the United States experience an episode of psychiatric illness during their lifetimes. Mood and anxiety disorders are the most common.
3. A significant number of people with psychiatric disorders also have a substance use disorder (SUD). SUDs are highest among those with antisocial or borderline personality disorders, bipolar illness, and schizophrenia.
4. Ask clients to share disorders or symptoms that they are experiencing. Then discuss the categories of psychiatric illness and types of symptoms associated with these illnesses (physical, cognitive, mood, behavioral).

    - *Mood disorders*: depression, mania, and mixed states.
    - *Anxiety disorders*: generalized anxiety, phobias, panic disorder, obsessive–compulsive disorder, and posttraumatic stress disorder.
    - *Psychotic disorders*: schizophrenia, schizoaffective disorder, and other psychotic disorders.
    - *Personality disorders*: antisocial, borderline, narcissistic, histrionic, paranoid, schizoid, avoidant, dependent, obsessive–compulsive, and "mixed."
    - *Other disorders*: eating disorders, compulsive gambling, impulse control, attention deficit, and adjustment disorders.

5. There are several different presentations of psychiatric illness.

    - *Single episode*: some people suffer only one episode of illness and once the symptoms remit they do not experience another episode.
    - *Recurrent episodes*: some people experience several episodes over time. They may function well between episodes. Episodes may occur years apart.

- *Chronic or persistent*: some clients experience some psychiatric symptoms more or less all the time. Even though they can get well and improve functioning, they may always have to cope with some symptoms.
- *Subsyndromal symptoms*: some clients experience psychiatric symptoms but do not meet criteria for a "diagnosis." These symptoms can cause personal suffering and impairment in life and often require treatment.

6. Stress that psychiatric disorders are best viewed as "no fault illnesses" and not a sign of "weakness." They are caused by a combination of factors such as:
    - *Biological factors*: these include hereditary predisposition, brain chemistry, and medical conditions. First-degree relatives of those with a psychiatric illness have increased odds for having one of these disorders. These disorders may also involve excesses or deficits of neurotransmitters in the brain. Medical problems, such as cancer or other diseases and substance abuse or addiction, can contribute to psychiatric disorders.
    - *Psychological factors*: these include defense mechanisms, personality, sensitivity to stress and how a person manages it, and a person's beliefs and cognitive style (e.g., how a person views himself, the world, and his problems).
    - *Social factors and life experiences*: these include family, social, and cultural influences, and exposure to trauma. For example, a traumatic injury, rape, assault, or exposure to a natural disaster, such as hurricane or flood, can contribute to psychiatric illness. So can exposure to persistent trauma such as violence, sexual abuse, or child abuse.
7. A continuum of care is needed to treat psychiatric disorders. This continuum includes inpatient psychiatric, residential, partial hospital, intensive outpatient, and outpatient treatment.
8. For chronic and recurrent conditions, ongoing involvement in "maintenance" treatment is needed. The client may return to see a therapist or psychiatrist every several months once stabilized from the acute symptoms of the disorders.
9. Somatic treatments include medications and electroshock therapy.
10. Ancillary services, including vocational rehabilitation or case management, are often needed.
11. Family involvement in treatment and recovery is helpful too. Families can learn what to do and what not to do to support their ill member. Family members can learn how to help themselves. In some instances, family members need help for their own psychiatric or substance use disorder.

Supporting Materials

Dennis C. Daley, *Dual Diagnosis Workbook: Recovery Strategies for Substance Use and Mental Health Disorders*, pp. 17–20. Independence, Missouri: Herald House/Independence Press, 2003.

Video: *Understanding Psychiatric Illness and Recovery*. Web site: *www.drdenniscdaley.com*.

PE Group Topic #3
Understanding Addiction

Objectives

1. Define addiction as a "no-fault" disease with specific symptoms.
2. Identify symptoms of addiction.
3. Identify biopsychosocial factors contributing to addiction.
4. Review treatment of addiction with an emphasis on the effectiveness of treatment.

Points for Discussion

1. More than 16 percent of adults in the United States will experience a substance use disorder (SUD) at some point in their lives.
2. A significant number of people with an SUD will also experience a psychiatric disorder at some point in their lives.
3. Ask clients to state their definitions of addiction. The American Medical Association classifies addiction as a disease. A disease is a "syndrome" with a cluster of specific symptoms. Similar to other medical and psychiatric disorders, addiction has a set of symptoms.
4. Ask clients to identify symptoms of addiction they have experienced. Provide additional examples that they fail to mention. Symptoms to review include:

   - *Excessive or inappropriate use of substances*: getting high or drunk and not being able to fulfill obligations at home, work, or with others; feeling like substances are needed in order to fit in with others or function at work or home; driving under the influence.

   - *Preoccupation with getting or using substances*: living mainly to get high on alcohol or drugs, substance use becomes too important in life, being obsessed with using.

   - *Tolerance changes*: needing more substance to get high or getting high much easier or with less substance than in the past.

   - *Having trouble cutting down or stopping*: not being able to control how much or how often substances are used, using more than planned.

   - *Withdrawal symptoms*: getting sick physically once the person cuts down or stops using (e.g., tremors, feeling nauseous, gooseflesh, a runny nose) or experiencing mental symptoms such as depression, anxiety, or agitation.

   - *Using to avoid or stop withdrawal symptoms*: using throughout the day to prevent withdrawal or using to stop withdrawal symptoms.

- *Using alcohol or other drugs even though they cause problems in life*: not taking a doctor's, therapist's, or other professional's advice to stop using because of problems that substances have caused in life.

- *Giving up important activities or losing friendships because of substance use*: stopping activities that once were important, giving up friends who don't get high, losing friends because substance use harms relationships.

- *Stopping use for a period of time (days, weeks, or months), only to go back again*: making temporary promises to quit, only to go back to getting high again; being unable to sustain abstinence.

- *Getting into trouble because of substance use*: losing jobs or being unable to find a job, getting arrested or having other legal problems, losing relationships or having trouble with family or friends, or having money problems.

- *Blackouts*: forgetting what one did or said while under the influence.

5. Ask clients to identify the factors they think contributed to their addiction. Ask if they have any family members with an addiction (current or past).

6. Review addiction as a biopsychosocial disease that is progressive and potentially fatal. Biological, psychological, and social factors all contribute to addiction.

7. Biological factors include the following:

    - *Hereditary predisposition*: first-degree relatives of addicted people have increased odds of becoming addicted.

    - *Brain chemistry*: repeated use of a substance can cause changes in the brain, leading to strong cravings. The pleasure felt from a drug induced high can surpass the pleasure felt from natural sources such as eating, sex, social interactions, sports, or accomplishments. Addictive drugs "hijack" the reward center of the brain.

    - *Physiology*: those who become addicted more easily develop a tolerance to the effects of substances. Some alcoholics, for example, initially develop a high tolerance for alcohol and are able to consume large quantities. Alcoholics are often unable to read their body cues that too much alcohol has been ingested.

8. Psychological or emotional factors include the following:

    - People with psychiatric illness are more vulnerable to developing an addiction compared to the general population.

    - Certain personality styles may increase a person's vulnerability to addiction.

    - Using alcohol or drugs to relax, escape, sleep, and deal with stress or uncomfortable emotions.

    - Exposure to a single trauma or repeated traumas over time (rape, violence, sexual abuse, child abuse, combat, or a natural disaster).

9. Social or cultural factors include the following:
   - Availability of alcohol or drugs.
   - Influence of peers and social groups.
   - Community norms governing substance use behavior.
10. Once an addiction develops, it takes on a life of its own. At this point, no external reason is needed for using substances as the addiction itself causes one to use.
11. Addiction is very treatable. Services for addiction include detoxification, short- and long-term rehabilitation, partial hospital, intensive outpatient, outpatient, and aftercare programs. Medications can help too.
12. Most people who participate in treatment improve. The key to benefiting from treatment is attending all sessions and not dropping out early.
13. The goals of treatment are to initiate and maintain abstinence, deal with problems contributing to or resulting from the addiction, and make personal and lifestyle changes.
14. For individuals with coexisting psychiatric illness, treatment of the psychiatric illness is necessary to experience the full benefits of recovery.
15. Support groups such as AA, NA, DRA, and others play a major role in the recovery of many individuals with addiction or dual disorders.

Supporting Materials

Dennis C. Daley, *Dual Diagnosis Workbook: Recovery Strategies for Substance Use and Mental Health Disorders*, pp. 25–28. Independence, Missouri: Herald House/Independence Press, 2003.

Dennis C. Daley, *Surviving Addiction Workbook: Practical Tips on Developing a Recovery Plan.* Holmes Beach, Florida: Learning Publications, 1999.

Dennis C. Daley and G. Alan Marlatt, *Managing Your Drug or Alcohol Problem: Client Guide.* San Antonio, Texas: Psychological Corporation, 1997a.

PE Group Topic #4
Effects of Dual Disorders

Objectives

1. Review the effects of disorders on medical, psychiatric, emotional, family, social, interpersonal, occupational, academic, legal, spiritual, and financial functioning.
2. Identify the effects of substance use on psychiatric symptoms.
3. Identify the effects of psychiatric illness on substance use.
4. Introduce the concept of "progression" of illness and that left untreated, either disorder can worsen over time.

Points for Discussion

1. Ask clients how their substance use has affected their lives and their psychiatric symptoms.
2. Ask clients how their psychiatric illness has affected their substance use or other problems in their lives.
3. Review problems associated with either or both disorders provided by clients. Discuss problems caused or worsened by either or both disorders related to:
   - Physical, medical or dental health, or sleep.
   - Diet and eating habits.
   - Sexual desire or behaviors.
   - Exercise habits and physical condition.
   - Mood or emotional control.
   - Suicidal or homicidal thoughts or actions.
   - Control over impulses and behaviors.
   - Relationships with family, friends, or coworkers.
   - Spirituality.
   - Work or school.
   - Lost opportunities or wasted talents or abilities.
   - Hobbies or leisure interests.
   - Financial condition.
   - Difficulty with the law or other legal problems.
4. State that either illness can worsen without treatment, a condition referred to as "progression."

5. Discuss positive effects of treatment based on outcome studies (for both substance use and psychiatric disorders). Treatment helps clients deal with problems associated with their disorders.

    - There is considerable evidence that psychiatric treatment helps reduce or eliminate psychiatric symptoms and improve functioning.

    - There is considerable evidence that treatment for an SUD helps clients stop or reduce substance use, reduce associated problems, and improve functioning.

    - Treatment also improves the quality of life.

6. Discuss how continued involvement in treatment provides an opportunity to deal with problems when they occur. This may help "small" problems from becoming serious ones.

Supporting Materials

Dennis C. Daley, *Double Recovery: Managing Your Substance Use and Mental Health Disorders.* Memphis, Tennessee: Foundations, 2004.

Dennis C. Daley, *Dual Diagnosis Workbook: Recovery Strategies for Substance Use and Mental Health Disorders*, pp. 29–31. Independence, Missouri: Herald House/Independence Press, 2003.

Video: *Double Trouble: Coping with Chemical Dependency and Mental Health Disorders.* Parts I and II. Wilmette, Illinois: Gerald T. Rogers Productions, phone: 1-800-227-9100; Web site: *www.gtrvideo.com.*

PE Group Topic #5
Medical Effects of Alcohol and Drugs

Objectives

1. Identify factors that mediate the effects of alcohol or other drugs on the body.
2. Identify physical and medical problems associated with substance use disorders.
3. Help clients identify medical effects of their substance use disorders.
4. Introduce clients to good physical and health care habits.

Points for Discussion

1. Substance use disorders are associated with many medical problems and diseases. The effects on a client depend on the following:
   - Types, frequency, quantity, and methods of use (for example, IV use, smoking).
   - Impurities in drugs or dirty needles, cotton, or rinsing water (for IV users).
   - How chemicals affect judgment and behavior. For example, poor judgment can lead to accidents while under the influence or involvement in high-risk behaviors such as unprotected sex, fights, or criminal acts. Clients who use expensive drugs like heroin or cocaine are more likely to engage in antisocial or criminal behaviors to get money to pay for their drugs.
   - Diet, overall health, and lifestyle.
2. Ask clients to identify physical and medical effects of their substance use disorders. Add to their list and review these effects:
   - Accidents, injuries, and close-to-death experiences.
   - Central nervous system problems (blackouts, memory problems, convulsions, slower reflexes).
   - Complications related to overdose or withdrawal.
   - Digestive system problems (cancers of the mouth, tongue, pharynx, and esophagus; ulcers, gastritis, pancreatitis).
   - Liver disease.
   - Acquiring or transmitting HIV or other infectious diseases.
   - Cardiovascular system problems (weakening of heart muscle, irregular heartbeat, heart pain, heart attack, stroke, and high blood pressure).
   - Respiratory system problems (lung disease and damage, infections).

- Sexual problems (diseases, problems with performance, problems with menstrual cycle).
- Worsening of existing medical conditions such as hypertension or diabetes.
- Loss of teeth or poor dental hygiene.
- Poor overall health including significant loss or gain of weight.

3. People with SUDs use medical services more frequently than others. The life span can be shortened due to the effects of substance use. More than 1 million people die every year from the direct and indirect effects of alcohol and drugs.
4. Tobacco and alcohol cause considerably more deaths and medical diseases than other substances.
5. Emphasize the importance of good physical and health care habits:
    - Getting regular examinations and help for existing medical or dental problems.
    - Adhering to a healthy diet and avoiding getting too hungry (remember HALT).
    - Getting sufficient rest, sleep, and exercise.
    - Using stress-reduction and stress-management activities (relaxation, meditation, prayer.).
    - Stopping the use of tobacco.

Supporting Materials

Dennis C. Daley, *Dual Diagnosis Workbook: Recovery Strategies for Substance Use and Mental Health Disorders*, pp. 42–44, Independence, Missouri: Herald House/Independence Press, 2003.

Independence Press, Hazelden, NIAAA, and NIDA have written materials and videos on medical effects of substances.

PE Group Topic #6
Withdrawal from Alcohol and Other Drugs

Objectives

1. Identify withdrawal symptoms of addictive substances.
2. Define acute and protracted withdrawal syndromes (also referred to as post-acute withdrawal).
3. Review when detoxification is needed, and identify methods to manage withdrawal symptoms.

Points for Discussion

1. Physical and emotional symptoms are associated with withdrawal from addictive substances. The types, intensity, and duration of symptoms depend on the severity of the addiction and the types, amounts, frequency, and methods of substance use.
2. Ask clients for personal examples of withdrawal symptoms experienced when reducing or stopping substance use. Define the early period as "acute withdrawal," and state that it lasts a few days or longer, depending on the substances a client has been using.
3. Ask clients for personal examples of symptoms experienced weeks into recovery. State that some people experience a "protracted or post-acute withdrawal" after they stop using substances. The body takes time to adjust to abstinence.
4. Specific withdrawal symptoms relate to the types of substances clients use. Withdrawal from alcohol or barbiturate dependence is the most dangerous due to the possibility of seizures.
5. Review withdrawal symptoms associated with alcohol and other drugs:
   - Shakes or tremors.
   - Anxiety or agitation.
   - Intense cravings for alcohol or other drugs.
   - Depression and sleep problems.
   - Runny nose, tearing eyes, gooseflesh.
   - Severe cramps, nausea, or feeling worn out.
   - Confusion or difficulty thinking clearly.
   - Convulsions or seizures.
6. Ask clients how they have managed their withdrawal symptoms in the past (most will report ingestion of alcohol or other drugs).

7. Detoxification is needed when clients cannot stop using on their own without health care risks or have coexisting medical or psychiatric disorders that may become complicated due to withdrawal symptoms.

8. Detoxification under the care of professionals in a hospital, residential, or ambulatory program can help the person safely withdrawal. Most detoxes last a few days.

9. Detoxification should be followed by continued care in a treatment and/or self-help program.

10. Review strategies to reduce and manage withdrawal symptoms:
    - Medications to safely and gradually withdraw from the addictive substance(s).
    - Rest and proper nutrition.
    - Supportive care of professionals.
    - Support from others (family, sponsor).
    - Gaining education about withdrawal symptoms and recovery.
    - Avoiding high-risk situations where substances are present (external "cues" can trigger withdrawal symptoms).
    - Getting rid of alcohol, drugs, or drug paraphernalia to reduce the chance of using substances to stop withdrawal symptoms.
    - Remembering that withdrawal is temporary.

Supporting Materials

Dennis C. Daley and G. Alan Marlatt, *Managing Your Drug or Alcohol Problem: Client Guide*. San Antonio, Texas: Psychological Corporation, 1997a.

Terence T. Gorski, *Learning to Live Again*. Independence, Missouri: Herald House/Independence Press. Phone: 1-800-767-8181; Web site: *www.relapse.org*.

Independence Press, Hazelden, NIAAA, and NIDA have written materials and videos on the effects of substances, including withdrawal symptoms.

PE Group Topic #7
Alcohol and Other Depressants

Objectives

1. Review the effects of alcohol and other depressants.
2. Identify medical problems associated with alcohol and other depressants.
3. Identify psychosocial and psychiatric problems associated with alcohol and other depressant abuse and dependence.

Points for Discussion

1. There are many different types of central nervous system (CNS) depressants. These include alcohol, hypnotics (barbiturates and barbiturate like drugs), and anti-anxiety drugs (tranquilizers) such as benzodiazepines.

2. Alcohol is widely used in our culture for many social events. Almost 14 percent of adults will develop alcohol abuse or dependence at some point in their lives.

   - Alcohol in beer has the same effect as alcohol in other beverages.
   - The legal limit for intoxication is a blood alcohol level (BAL) of .80 or .10 in most states. The higher the BAL, the greater the likelihood of an accident.
   - If a person does not "feel drunk" after consuming a large quantity of alcohol, it is due to a high tolerance. Even if a client does not feel drunk, judgment, behavior, and ability are impaired. Some people with a high BAL feel "normal" and believe they can drive safely.
   - Mixing alcohol with other depressant drugs potentiates their effects.
   - Alcohol use in small qualities can lead to poor judgment, causing a person to say or do things that would not occur if not drinking.
   - Some people believe alcohol gives a person "courage" to say what is really on the mind. In reality, the "truth" that comes out can be distorted or exaggerated. Mild irritation may be expressed as passionate hatred. Attraction may falsely be stated as deep love.
   - Victims and perpetrators of homicide and other forms of violence are often under the influence of alcohol during the episode.

3. CNS depressant drugs are used to treat medical and psychiatric disorders. Some of these drugs are more addictive than others.

4. These drugs have various effects and are dangerous when taken in large doses; they can cause death by coma or convulsions. Withdrawal is more severe than with other drugs.

5. Symptoms associated with excessive use of depressant drugs or withdrawal include anxiety, depression, sleep disturbance, impaired judgment, impaired coordination, slurred speech, tremors, weakness, sweating, increased pulse rate, nausea and vomiting, memory loss or blackouts, seizures, and confusion.

6. Hundreds of thousands of people die each year from the effects of alcohol.

7. Due to the effects of alcohol or other depressants, poor diet or health care practices, or concurrent use of tobacco, the risk of medical and psychiatric problems is higher among alcoholics compared to the general population.

8. Elicit examples of client's medical problems caused by their substance use:
    - Ulcer disease, liver disease, and heart disease.
    - Gastritis (inflammation of the stomach).
    - Pancreatitis (inflammation of the pancreas).
    - Cancers of the esophagus, stomach, head and neck, and lungs.
    - Organic brain diseases.
    - Peripheral neuropathy (deterioration of peripheral nerves to hands or feet).
    - Sexual disorders.
    - Trauma caused by accidents, head injury, or toxic overdoses.

9. Elicit examples of psychosocial problems caused or worsened by substance use:
    - Accidents and impaired ability to drive or operate machinery.
    - Violence and other antisocial behaviors.
    - Anxiety and panic symptoms.
    - Depression, suicidal feelings, or actual attempts.
    - Work, school, family, legal, financial, or other spiritual problems.

Supporting Materials

Independence Press, Hazelden, NIAAA, NCADI, and AA World Services have videos and/or written materials on alcohol problems and recovery.

PE Group Topic #8
Cocaine and Other Stimulants

Objectives

1. Review the effects of cocaine and other stimulant drugs.
2. Identify medical problems associated with cocaine and other stimulants.
3. Identify psychosocial and psychiatric problems associated with cocaine and other stimulants.

Points for Discussion

1. Stimulants include cocaine, amphetamines, caffeine, and nicotine.
2. Stimulant drugs are prescribed to treat narcolepsy, attention deficit disorder with hyperactivity, obesity, and depression. Excessive use can cause symptoms that mimic psychiatric symptoms.
3. These drugs can be taken in the form of pills, injected with a needle, or smoked in the form of freebase cocaine or crack.
4. Cocaine is sometimes mixed with heroin and injected. Many people use alcohol to help cope with the "crash" when coming off a cocaine or speed binge.
5. Crack/cocaine is a cheap form of smokeable cocaine that can be bought in the form of "rocks" for as little as $3 to $5.
6. Stimulants release neurotransmitters, such as norepinephrine, from nerve cells. These can cause a decrease in reuptake of the neurotransmitter dopamine.
7. These drugs cause feelings of euphoria, increase energy, decrease fatigue, decrease the need for sleep, decrease appetite, and sometimes increase sexual feelings and sexual energy. Medical problems associated with stimulants include the following:
   - An increase in the heart rate that can cause an elevation of blood pressure. Elevated blood pressure can cause hemorrhaging in the cranium.
   - Increase in heart rate that can cause cardiac fibrillation, respiratory arrest, and death.
   - Pulmonary problems such as bronchitis.
   - Contaminated needles may cause complications such as hepatitis, abscesses, AIDS virus, or endocarditis.
   - Damage to the nasal septum (for clients who snort cocaine).
   - Damage to an unborn fetus in pregnant women.

8. Cocaine and other stimulants can cause a withdrawal syndrome. Symptoms include depression, fatigue, unpleasant dreams, sleep disturbance, increased appetite, and psychomotor agitation or retardation.

9. These drugs may cause serious psychiatric and psychosocial problems. Ask clients for examples and add additional ones such as the following:

    - Depression, suicidal feelings, and attempts.
    - Accidents.
    - Violence, antisocial behaviors, and impulsive behaviors.
    - Psychosis, including paranoia.
    - Panic symptoms.
    - Work, family, legal, financial, and other problems.

10. Many people with stimulant addiction also have a serious problem with alcohol or other drugs.

11. Abstinence from alcohol and all drugs is important for recovery to progress. Continuing to drink alcohol or smoke pot significantly raises the risk of relapse to cocaine use.

Supporting Materials

Independence Press, Hazelden, NCADI, NIDA, and NA have written materials and videos on cocaine/stimulant problems and recovery from drug addiction.

Video: *Recovery from Crack/Cocaine Addiction*. Wilmette, Illinois: Gerald T. Rogers Productions. Phone: 1-800-227-9100; Web site: *www.gtrvideo.com*.

PE Group Topic #9
Heroin and Other Opiates

Objectives
1. Review the effects of heroin and other opiates.
2. Identify medical problems associated with these drugs.
3. Identify psychosocial and psychiatric problems associated with opiate abuse and dependence.

Points for Discussion
1. Opiates include street drugs, like heroin or opium, or prescription narcotics, such as Methadone, Dilaudid, Percodan, Darvon, Vicodin, and Oxycontin.
2. Opiates can be ingested by using a needle, snorting, smoking, or in pill form. Some addicts mix cocaine with heroin ("speedball").
3. Prescribed opiates are used to reduce or control pain or as cough suppressants.
4. Effects of opiates depend on the types and amounts used, methods of use, and psychological state of the user.
5. Opiates are dangerous when taken in large doses and can cause death by coma.
6. Symptoms associated with excessive use of opiate drugs or withdrawal include depression, nausea, vomiting, muscle aches, runny nose, yawning, tearing eyes, sweating, tremors, sleep and appetite disturbance, weakness, fever, chills, cramping and abdominal pain, diarrhea, gooseflesh, and strong drug cravings. Withdrawal is not as severe or life threatening as alcohol or barbiturates.
7. Opiate addicts die from overdoses, suicides, homicides, and medical problems such as AIDs caused by sharing dirty cotton, rinsing water, or needles.
8. Elicit examples of medical problems caused or worsened by client's opiate drug use such as:
   - HIV infections and AIDS
   - Skin and muscle abscesses and infections
   - Liver disease
   - Tetanus or malaria
   - Gastric ulcers
   - Kidney failure
   - Endocarditis

- Heart arrhythmias
- Sexual dysfunctions

9. Elicit examples of psychosocial or psychiatric problems caused or worsened by their opiate addiction such as:
   - Drug overdoses
   - Depression, suicidal feelings, or actual attempts
   - Antisocial and criminal behaviors, including violence, to get money to buy drugs
   - Work, family, legal, financial, spiritual, and other problems

10. Many opiate addicts abuse other drugs or transfer their addiction to alcohol or cocaine once they stop using opiates.

11. Heroin is "cut" with adulterants that can be dangerous when ingested.

12. Opiate addicts unable to get and stay drug free with rehabilitation programs, counseling, and/or NA may benefit from methadone maintenance (MM). MM is a treatment in which methadone "replaces" the other opiate drugs allowing the affected individual to function. MM is usually offered in conjunction with counseling.

13. Other medications for opiate addiction include buprenorphine and naltrexone. Buprenorphine (Buprenex) is used to ease withdrawal and as a replacement drug in maintenance therapy. Naltrexone (Trexan) blocks the euphoric high of opiate drugs so the addicted person does not feel the usual "high" from opiates.

Supporting Materials

Hazelden, NIDA, NIAAA, NCADI, and Narcotics Anonymous have written materials and/or videos on opiate drugs and recovery from opiate addiction.

PE Group Topic #10
Psychosocial Effects of Substance Disorders

Objectives

1. Identify psychosocial problems caused or worsened by substance use disorders.
2. Help clients identify specific psychosocial problems experienced as a result of their substance use disorders.
3. Help clients identify strategies to cope with these problems.

Points for Discussion

1. Substance use disorders (SUDs) are associated with many psychological, psychiatric, family, interpersonal, social, academic, occupational, legal, spiritual, and financial problems. SUDs cause new problems or make existing ones worse.
2. Elicit examples of problems caused or worsened by substance use. Use examples of clients and add new ones to summarize problems associated with SUDs, methods of use (e.g., dirty needles), or a lifestyle centered around substance use. Problems include the following:
   - *Health*: injuries, infectious diseases, medical disorders, dental problems, sleep problems, and weight loss.
   - *Psychiatric*: acute and chronic use of substances can cause cognitive, mood-related, physical or behavioral symptoms. Psychiatric disorders are more common among those with alcohol (37 percent) or drug abuse or dependence (53 percent) compared to the general population (22 percent).
   - *Psychological*: judgment, motivation, emotional control, memory, self-esteem, and control over behavior are affected by SUDs.
   - *Family*: SUDs contribute to divorce and family breakups and have adverse effects on family members, including children. Children of substance abusers are more likely than other kids to have an SUD, psychiatric illness, academic, or behavioral problems. Many people with SUDs become disconnected from parents, siblings, children, and other relatives. Much heartache is caused in families by substance problems.
   - *Interpersonal and social*: relationships can be harmed or lost and non-substance social activities may be given up.
   - *Occupational and academic*: SUDs may lead to underfunctioning at school or work, an inability to find or keep a job, poor grades, or flunking out of school.
   - *Legal*: SUDs contribute to legal and criminal behaviors. Many people are incarcerated for crimes caused by the effects of substances or to get money to pay for drugs.

- *Spiritual*: shame, guilt, feeling empty, and becoming disconnected from loved ones or church are common spiritual problems associated with SUDs.
- *Financial*: SUDs can lead to debt, failure to pay bills, and inability to meet living expenses.

3. Discuss the importance of resolving these problems as recovery progresses. Emphasize the need to limit the number of problems addressed in early recovery so that clients do not feel overwhelmed.
4. Ask clients to choose one problem caused by their addiction that they would like to begin working on.
5. Ask clients to identify cognitive and behavioral coping strategies that can help them deal with this problem. Ask other clients for additional ideas on coping strategies to manage the problems discussed.

Supporting Materials

Dennis C. Daley, *Dual Diagnosis Workbook: Recovery Stratgies for Substance Use and Mental Health Disorders*, pp. 29–31. Independence, Missouri: Herald House/Independence Press, 2003.

Dennis C. Daley and G. Alan Marlatt, *Managing Your Drug or Alcohol Problem: Practical Tips on Developing a Recovery Plan*, pp. 17–22. Holmes Beach, Florida: Learning Publications, 1999.

Independence Press, Hazelden, NIDA, NIAAA, AA, and NA have written materials and/or videos on psychosocial effects of substances and recovery from addiction.

PE Group Topic #11
How to Use Treatment: Keys to Successful Recovery

Objectives

1. Identify client's expectations of treatment and recovery.
2. Review the importance of taking an "active" role in recovery and taking responsibility for change.
3. Identify the benefits and limitations of professional treatment.
4. Review attitudes and behaviors that promote a positive recovery.

Points for Discussion

1. It is important for clients to have realistic expectations regarding treatment and recovery. Unrealistic expectations, especially those that are too high, will set clients up to fail, feel frustrated, or feel disappointed.
2. Ask clients to discuss expectations of professional treatment.
   - What do they hope to get from treatment?
   - How do they see their role in treatment and recovery?
   - How do they view their responsibility in terms of treatment compliance and testing out new behaviors?
3. Stress the importance of clients taking an "active" role in treatment. This means working with their treatment team to do the following:
   - Identify problems and goals.
   - Identify strategies to change and reach their goals.
   - Practice and implement change strategies.
   - Change ineffective strategies.
4. Review how treatment can help and review limitations of treatment and the professionals providing it. For example:
   - A therapist will not always be available for phone discussions and may not be able to give counseling appointments as often as clients would like.
   - Even medications may have a limited impact on psychiatric symptoms. It is not easy to find the right medicine.
   - Changing a therapist or doctor is not always advisable. The client should not "fire" a doctor or therapist without discussing the reasons and getting input from an objective person.

5. Discuss attitudes and behaviors that aid long-term recovery such as the following:
   - Being honest with professionals and sponsor about problems, struggles, feelings, and thoughts.
   - Being realistic, patient, and persistent regarding change.
   - Making a commitment to recovery.
   - Attending all treatment sessions and being on time.
   - Being self-reflective.
   - Setting realistic goals for change.
   - Sharing goals with others and asking for their feedback.
   - Knowing when and how to ask others for help and support.
   - Applying coping strategies to deal with problems.
   - Participating in AA, NA, DRA, or other support groups; using a sponsor.
   - Allowing room for mistakes and learning from them.
   - Evaluating progress regularly and changing the treatment plan as needed.
   - Developing "inner resources" and learning ways to help oneself.

Supporting Materials

Dennis C. Daley, *Double Recovery: Managing Your Substance Use and Mental Health Disorders*. Memphis, Tennessee: Foundations, 2004.

Dennis C. Daley, *Dual Diagnosis Workbook: Recovery Strategies for Substance Use and Mental Health Disorders*, pp 35–36. Independence, Missouri: Herald House/Independence Press, 2003.

Video: *Understanding Psychiatric Illness and Recovery*. Web site: *www.drdenniscdaley.com*.

PE Group Topic #12
Phases of Recovery

Objectives

1. Introduce clients to "phases of recovery" from dual disorders.
2. Identify key issues for each of the phases of recovery.

Points for Discussion

1. There are different phases of recovery for dual disorders. Each phase has specific issues related to the psychiatric or substance use disorders. These phases are "rough" guidelines. Not everyone progresses through them at the same pace or in the same way. The severity of the illnesses and the client's motivation affect how they will progress through these phases.
2. Review each of these phases to summarize and discuss key themes.

Phase 1—Transition and Engagement (up to several weeks)

- Entry into treatment may result from an involuntary commitment or pressure from family or others to get help.
- Become engaged in treatment and accept the need for ongoing involvement in treatment.
- Recognize an inability to control substance use and that substances can mask, trigger, or worsen psychiatric symptoms.
- Recognize and accept the psychiatric disorder and the need for treatment. Understand that an untreated disorder will interfere with recovery from addiction.
- Recognize ambivalence about recovery and making changes.
- Invite the family or significant others to treatment.

Phase 2—Stabilization (weeks or longer)

- Stabilize from acute psychiatric symptoms.
- Get alcohol and drugs out of system and adjust to being substance free.
- Become educated about the dual disorders, the role of therapy and medications, and the role of self-help programs.
- Accept the disorders and need for treatment and involvement in recovery.
- Develop trust in the treatment team.

- Learn to cope with thoughts of using or cravings for alcohol or drugs.
- Learn to manage symptoms of the psychiatric illness.
- Participate in self-help programs.
- Strengthen motivation to recover.
- Develop a problem list to work on during recovery.
- Accept the need for abstinence from alcohol, street drugs, and non-prescribed drugs as the path to take in recovery.
- Continue family involvement in treatment.

Phase 3—Early Recovery (three to six months)

- Continue work from Phase 2 (e.g., managing persistent symptoms).
- Avoid or minimize exposure to people, places, events, and things that represent a relapse risk for addiction.
- Learn to cope with pressures from others to use substances and situations that in the past led to use.
- Challenge addictive and inaccurate or negative thinking.
- Accept that medications can reduce symptoms but other changes are necessary for recovery to progress.
- Change behaviors, especially ones that caused difficulties in the past.
- Build structure and regularity into daily life to keep busy, stay focused on recovery, get involved in enjoyable leisure activities, and limit free time.
- Continue family work and learn about the impact of the dual disorders and behaviors on the family.
- Continue involvement in support groups and work with a sponsor.
- Address guilt and shame issues.

Phase 4—Middle Recovery (six to twelve months)

- Continue work from Phase 3.
- Increase self-disclosure about inner thoughts, feelings, and problems.
- Make amends to family and others hurt by behaviors.
- Accept that some relationships cannot be fixed or salvaged.
- Improve communication and strengthen relationships.
- Focus on spirituality issues.
- Continue improving cognitive and behavioral coping strategies to deal with negative or upsetting thoughts and feelings and problems.

- Identify and manage warning signs of relapse of all disorders.
- Monitor recovery on a daily basis.
- Deal with trauma or family of origin issues if needed to heal past emotional wounds.

Phase 5—Late Recovery (a year or more)
- Continue work from Phase 4.
- Continue developing positive values and meaning in life.
- Increase awareness of "inner self" (defenses, personality traits, values, strengths, and vulnerabilities).
- Gain greater understanding of "past" influences on current behaviors, values, and relationships.
- Broaden support group involvement (e.g., ACOA or survivor groups).
- Focus on changing character defects (personality traits).
- Focus more on "lifestyle balancing" so that attention is directed to all areas of life—recovery, work, relationships, love, fun, and spirituality.

Phase 6—Maintenance (ongoing)
- This is an ongoing phase where the work of recovery continues with less reliance on a therapist or sponsor.
- More attention is directed toward "giving away" what one learned in recovery by sponsoring others or serving the greater good of society.
- There is no time limit as some people continue involvement in treatment, self-help programs, or a self-management program of change for an indefinite period of time.
- Lapses or relapses to substance use, recurrences of psychiatric symptoms or other life setbacks are dealt with as they occur. A relapse does not mean that the client has failed or needs to start recovery over again.

Supporting Materials

Dennis C. Daley, *Double Recovery: Managing Your Substance Use and Mental Health Disorders*. Memphis, Tennessee: Foundations, 2004.

Dennis C. Daley, *Dual Diagnosis Workbook: Recovery Strategies for Substance Use and Mental Health Disorders*, pp. 58–66. Independence, Missouri: Herald House/Independence Press, 2003.

PE Group Topic #13
Developing a Problem List

Objectives

1. Review how to develop a problem list and treatment goals.
2. Help clients incorporate substance related, psychiatric, and other important lifestyle problems on the master problem list.
3. Review problems associated with dual disorders.
4. Help clients identify personal strengths and resiliencies.

Points for Discussion

1. Ask clients why they came to treatment. Their reasons may include psychiatric or substance use disorders or problems associated with either or both disorders.
2. Briefly review problems associated with dual disorders.
   - Motivational
   - Cognitive
   - Emotional
   - Interpersonal
   - Social
   - Spiritual
   - Legal
   - Financial
   - Medical
3. Discuss the importance of prioritizing problems and limiting the focus on just a few in early recovery.
4. Emphasize that during the early stages of recovery the main emphasis is on stabilizing acute psychiatric symptoms and getting sober.
5. Discuss the importance of sobriety. Discuss the impact of continued substance use on psychiatric recovery. Substance use can do the following:
   - Mask, trigger, or worsen psychiatric symptoms.
   - Lower motivation to change.
   - Have a negative impact on adherence to treatment and recovery.
   - Lower the effectiveness of medications or cause dangerous interactions.

6. Every client has personal strengths and resiliencies. Ask clients to identify their strengths and resiliencies that can aid their recovery such as the following:
    - Positive qualities such as being friendly, loving, sociable, kind, altruistic, committed, resourceful, or assertive.
    - Talents such as athletic, musical, artistic, mechanical, or other abilities.
    - Faith in God or belief in a Higher Power.
    - Positive relationships with family, friends, AA/NA/DRA members, professional caregivers, or others.
    - Positive attitudes about recovery and willingness to work hard.
    - Positive attitudes about life.
    - Stable living, job, or economic situation.
    - Ability to bounce back from adversity and learn from problems or personal suffering.

Supporting Materials

Dennis C. Daley, *Dual Diagnosis Workbook: Recovery Strategies for Substand Use and Mental Health Disorders*, pp. 32–34. Independence, Missouri: Herald House/Independence Press, 2003.

PE Group Topic #14
Setting Treatment Goals

Objectives

1. Review the importance of setting goals in treatment.
2. Review the importance of short-, medium-, and long-term goals.
3. Help clients prioritize their goals.
4. Help clients develop plans to reach one goal.

Points for Discussion

1. Define goals as statements about what a person wants to achieve (i.e., to learn, do, accomplish). Goals imply action toward an end and are best described with "action verbs." Goals may be related to recovery (e.g., managing the disorders) or to life (e.g., getting a job, developing a new relationship).

2. Ask clients why it is important to set goals in relation to the problems that led to treatment.
   - Goals make treatment an active process by providing a focus for change.
   - Goals provide structure and a way to reach specific ends that are desirable.
   - Goals are a way to judge progress toward a desired end.
   - The process of working toward a goal can be as important as the goal itself.
   - Goals give a sense of direction and provide hope.

3. Ask clients for examples of goals such as the following:
   - Eliminate, reduce, or manage specific psychiatric symptoms.
   - Get sober and learn to manage the substance use disorder.
   - Learn information about a specific disorder, problem, or topic (e.g., addiction, anxiety, mood disorders, spirituality).
   - Learn skills to manage the disorders or problems such as anger or relationship conflicts.

4. Define short-, medium-, and long-term goals as follows:
   - Short-term: fewer than three months.
   - Medium-term: four to twelve months.
   - Long-term: one year or longer.

5. State the importance of having an "action plan" to follow to reach one's goals.

6. Ask for examples of "action plans" that clients have followed in pursuing goals. Emphasize the need to have several coping strategies rather than just one.

   - *Cognitive strategies*: changing thoughts and beliefs, reflecting on oneself, recovery and life, and thinking through problems.

   - *Behavioral strategies*: changing how one acts or copes with problems.

   - *Interpersonal strategies*: using help and support from others, improving communication and relationships.

   - *Physical/lifestyle strategies*: changing health care habits, exercising, following a diet, or changing lifestyle.

   - *Emotional strategies*: changing how one manages feelings or mood states.

   - *Spiritual strategies*: using a Higher Power, prayer, meditation, forgiveness, helping others, or focusing on contributing to the good of society.

7. Stress the importance of taking an active role in identifying and setting goals, developing action plans, and putting these plans into action, if goals. Discuss the importance of "walking the walk," not just "talking the talk" of recovery.

8. Discuss the need to practice new behaviors and accept that mistakes may be made, and it may take time to make successful changes.

9. Elicit examples of successful changes that clients have made. Discuss what they think was involved in making these changes (e.g., putting forth effort, taking time to change, having a plan, using support from others, and learning from mistakes).

Supporting Materials

Dennis C. Daley, *Dual Diagnosis Workbook: Recovery Strategies for Substance Use and Mental Health Disorders*, pp. 35–36. Independence, Missouri: Herald House/Independence Press, 2003.

PE Group Topic #15
Advantages of Recovery

Objectives

1. Review advantages and disadvantages of sobriety.
2. Identify advantages and disadvantages associated with recovery.

Points for Discussion

1. There are advantages and disadvantages associated with giving up alcohol and drugs and initiating a program of recovery from substance use and psychiatric disorders. Points to emphasize and discuss include the following:

   - It is not easy to stop using substances and stay sober, especially in the early phases of recovery. A feeling of "loss" or "grief" is common with abstinence.
   - Many clients in early recovery are ambivalent about sobriety. A part of them wants to continue using substances while another part wants to get sober.
   - Clients need to acknowledge and accept they have an "addicted side" that wants to use substances and a "healthy side" that wants sobriety.
   - Acknowledging this ambivalence helps clients become able to focus on the advantages of giving up alcohol or drugs and changing.

2. Ask clients what they will miss about not using substances or living a lifestyle that is no longer centered on substance use.

3. Discuss the positive aspects of sobriety and getting help for the psychiatric disorder. These include improvements in:

   - Physical health.
   - Psychiatric status or mental health.
   - Psychological health: better control over emotions, thinking, impulses, and behaviors; improved self-esteem.
   - Cognitive abilities: think more clearly, solve problems.
   - Family and social relationships.
   - Ability to work or attend school.
   - Spiritual health.
   - Financial situation.
   - Quality of life.

4. Discuss the advantages and disadvantages associated with involvement in an ongoing program of recovery. Points to emphasize and discuss include the following:
   - Recovery requires patience, discipline, and hard work.
   - Recovery has rough spots; it is not always easy and at times one may want to give up or question the ability to change.
   - A program of dual recovery helps the client address both types of disorders and make changes.
   - Although there may be disadvantages, these are outweighed by the potential advantages of recovery.
5. Elicit personal examples of advantages or disadvantages clients have experienced or expect to experience in recovery.
6. Ask clients how they have used the support of other people or organizations (AA, NA, DRA, Church) to aid their recovery.

Supporting Materials

Dennis C. Daley, *Dual Diagnosis Workbook: Recovery Strategies for Substance Use and Mental Health Disorders*, pp. 39–41. Independence, Missouri: Herald House/Independence Press, 2003.

PE Group Topic #16
Denial in Addiction and Psychiatric Illness

Objectives

1. Discuss the psychological defense of denial.
2. Identify specific ways denial of illness shows.
3. Identify effects of denial of either or both disorders.
4. Review strategies to accept the dual disorders.

Points for Discussion

1. Discuss psychological defenses with a focus on denial. Give examples of denial. State that these defenses are "unconscious" and occur out of awareness.
2. Denial is common in substance use and psychiatric disorders. It is the refusal to believe a painful reality in life and serves to "protect" a person from the anxiety associated with facing the truth about a serious problem.
3. Families and others can deny either or both disorders. They have difficulty accepting the reality of psychiatric illness, addiction, or both in a loved one.
4. Elicit examples of denial of psychiatric illness:
    - Blaming problems on bad luck, bad breaks, bad genes, or bad friends instead of acknowledging a psychiatric illness.
    - Minimizing the seriousness of the psychiatric disorder (e.g., seeing oneself as having a bad case of the blues instead of a depressive illness).
    - Refusing to believe one has a psychiatric illness because one holds a job, takes care of a family, or still functions fairly well in various areas of life.
    - Blaming psychiatric symptoms on alcohol or other drugs.
5. Elicit examples of denial of the substance use disorder (SUD):
    - Minimizing the problem because substances are not used every day or clients do not always lose control and get drunk or high when using.
    - Believing substance use is due to the psychiatric disorder.
    - Acknowledging the SUD, but refusing help.
    - Failure to accept abstinence as a goal or agreeing to give up the "main" substance of abuse but using "other" substances (i.e., giving up cocaine or heroin, but continuing to use alcohol or marijuana).
6. Discuss effects of denial of either or both disorders such as the following:

- Ending up in a psychiatric hospital involuntarily.
- Experiencing negative health, legal, family, or social consequences.
- Inability to recover from one illness due to denial of the other.

7. Discuss recovery strategies to work through denial.
   - Reviewing the symptoms, behaviors, and effects of psychiatric illness on self and others. Stress the importance of clients knowing their diagnoses.
   - Reviewing patterns of substance use, behaviors, and effects on self and others. Stress the importance of knowing the diagnoses.
   - Getting feedback from professionals, family members, or others regarding diagnoses, behaviors, or symptoms related to the disorders.

Supporting Materials

Dennis C. Daley, *Dual Diagnosis Workbook: Recovery Strategies for Substance Use and Mental Health Disorders*, pp. 46–53. Independence, Missouri: Herald House/Independence Press, 2003.

Dennis C. Daley, *Working through Denial*. Center City, Minnesota: Hazelden, 1998.

Terence T. Gorski, *Denial Management Counseling Workbook*. Independence, Missouri: Herald House/Independence Press, 2000.

PE Group Topic #17
Roadblocks in Recovery

Objectives

1. Review common roadblocks or barriers to recovery.
2. Have clients identify their personal roadblocks to recovery.
3. Have clients develop strategies to work through roadblocks so they do not sabotage the recovery process.
4. Reinforce the importance of staying involved in treatment and support groups when motivation wavers.

Points for Discussion

1. There are many barriers or roadblocks that can interfere with recovery. Ask clients for examples of their personal attitude, personality, relationship, or lifestyle factors that can impede recovery.
2. Use their examples and add others to review the following categories of roadblocks to change.
   - *Attitude and motivation roadblocks* such as low motivation to change, difficulty accepting either or both disorders, or not caring about recovery.
   - *Personality roadblocks* such as being stubborn and not letting others help, giving up too easily when things are difficult, or difficulty opening up.
   - *Relationship roadblocks* such as living with a person who gets high or not having a confidant or someone to confide in.
   - *Lifestyle roadblocks* such as lack of structure or routine in daily life, failure to plan for the future, or having no direction in life.
   - *Treatment participation roadblocks* such as missing counseling sessions, dropping out early, or failure to take medications as prescribed.
3. Emphasize that awareness of personal roadblocks puts clients in a position to begin working through them.
4. Ask clients to each identify one roadblock and specific ways to work through this roadblock.
5. Emphasize commonalities in these recovery roadblocks and positive coping strategies. Add additional coping strategies to ones provided by clients as the discussion unfolds.
6. Discuss the importance of staying in treatment even when clients want to drop out or struggle with their motivation.

7. Discuss the importance of continuing AA, NA, and/or DRA meetings even when clients want to stop attending or struggle with their motivation.

8. Discuss the importance of using support from other people to help overcome recovery roadblocks.

Supporting Materials

Dennis C. Daley, *Dual Diagnosis Workbook: Recovery Strategies for Substance Use and Mental Health Disorders*, pp. 54–57. Independence, Missouri: Herald House/Independence Press, 2003.

Dennis C. Daley and G. Alan Marlatt, *Managing Your Drug or Alcohol Problem*, pp. 35–38. San Antonio, Texas: Psychological Corporation, 1997a.

Video: *How to Sabotage Your Treatment*. Wilmette, Illinois: Gerald T. Rogers Productions. Phone: 1-800-227-9100; Web site: *www.gtrvideo.com*.

PE Group Topic #18
Recovery from Dual Disorders

Objectives

1. Review recovery as a process of ongoing management of the dual disorders.
2. Introduce recovery as motivation plus information plus skills plus a program of change (treatment and self-help).
3. Review physical, psychological, family, interpersonal, social, and spiritual aspects of recovery.
4. Identify benefits of recovery.

Points for Discussion

1. Ask clients to define recovery. Discuss recovery as a long-term "process" that involves abstinence, learning new coping strategies, and changing lifestyle.
2. Specific types of treatment are needed, depending on the psychiatric and substance use disorders that the clients are experiencing.
    - *Therapy or counseling*: there are a number of different therapies for addiction, psychiatric illness, or both such as interpersonal, supportive, cognitive behavioral, dual disorders counseling, relapse prevention, and skills training.
    - *Family treatment*: there are various types of couples and family treatment. Some are for specific disorders; others are used with any type of illness.
    - *Special programs*: day hospital, psychiatric rehabilitation, or intensive outpatient programs that involve combination treatments (individual, group, and social activities).
    - *Medications*: for psychiatric illness, addiction, or both.
    - *Self-help programs*: for psychiatric illness, addiction, or both. Programs are available for clients and their families.
    - *Other services*: vocational rehabilitation, GED or educational programs, case management, parenting classes
3. Emphasize the need to develop "internal" motivation for change.
4. Ask clients to identify one change to make. Use their answers to provide a bio-psycho-social-spiritual framework for recovery.
    - Physical recovery
    - Psychological recovery
    - Family recovery

- Interpersonal recovery (relationships and communication)
- Spiritual recovery
- Financial recovery

5. Ask clients to discuss the length of time they think they need to stay involved in professional treatment and/or self-help programs. Emphasize the importance of dealing both with short-term and long-term recovery issues.

6. Ask clients to identify potential benefits of recovery in the following areas:
   - Physical and medical (e.g., improved health).
   - Psychological (e.g., improved emotional control, improvement in problem-solving ability).
   - Family (e.g., better family relationships).
   - Social and interpersonal (e.g., improved relationships).
   - Spiritual (e.g., reduced shame and guilt, increased meaning in life).
   - Legal (e.g., resolution of legal problems).
   - Occupational (e.g., better attendance or productivity).
   - Financial (e.g., less debt, paying bills on time).

Supporting Materials

Dennis C. Daley, *Coping with Dual Disorders*. Center City, Minnesota: Hazelden, 1993.

Dennis C. Daley, *Double Recovery: Managing Your Substance Use and Mental Health Disorder*. Memphis, Tennessee: Foundations, 2004.

Dennis C. Daley, *Dual Diagnosis Workbook: Recovery Strategies for Substance Use and Mental Health Disorders*, pp. 58–66. Independence, Missouri: Herald House/Independence Press, 2003.

The Dual Disorders Recovery Book. Center City, Minnesota: Hazelden. Phone: 1-800-257-7810; Fax: 651-213-4411; Web site: *www.hazelden.org*.

PE Group Topic #19
Managing Cravings for Alcohol or Drugs

Objectives

1. Define cues, triggers, or precipitants of substance craving.
2. Identify external and internal precipitants of cravings.
3. Review strategies to manage cravings

Points for Discussion

1. Ask clients to define and describe cravings for alcohol or drugs.
   - How do cravings show in physical symptoms?
   - How do cravings show in their thoughts?
   - How do cravings show in their behaviors?
2. Ask clients to identify factors that trigger their cravings.
   - People, places, events, and things (external).
   - Thoughts, feelings, or physical pain (internal).
3. Discuss levels of intensity of cravings (from mild to severe). The level of craving will determine coping strategies to use.
4. Review how drugs "hijack" the reward system of the brain, which results in substances bringing more pleasure than food, sex, or other activities.
5. One result of this hijacking is the susceptibility to "cravings" when experiencing memories of substance use or exposed to external triggers.
6. This hijacking helps to partially explain the "compulsion" to use substances despite the damage they cause.
7. Discuss the importance of using multiple strategies to manage cravings since one strategy may not work in every instance of a craving.
8. Review coping strategies to manage cravings:
   - Recognizing and labeling the craving
   - Talking about the craving with a sponsor or confidante
   - Going to a self-help meeting such as AA, NA, or DRA and talking to others to find what they have done to manage their cravings
   - Talking oneself through the craving
   - Accepting that the craving will pass in time

- Redirecting activity to distract oneself temporarily from the craving
- Writing thoughts and feelings in a journal
- Getting rid of alcohol, drugs, and paraphernalia (external triggers)
- Avoiding high-risk people, places, events, and things when possible
- Praying or using a Higher Power
- Reading recovery literature
- Writing in a journal

Supporting Materials

Dennis C. Daley, *Dual Diagnosis Workbook: Recovery Strategies for Substance Use and Mental Health Disorders*, pp. 67–71. Independence, Missouri: Herald House/Independence Press, 2003.

Video: *Coping with Cravings and Thoughts of Using*. Wilmette, Illinois: Gerald T. Rogers Productions. Phone: 1-800-227-9100; Web site: *www.gtrvideo.com*.

PE Group Topic #20
Managing People, Places, Events, and Things

Objectives

1. Define the concept of "high-risk people, places, events, and things."
2. Help clients identify their own high-risk people, places, events, and things.
3. Review strategies to manage high-risk people, places, events, and things.

Points for Discussion

1. All clients have "high-risk people, places, events, and things" that can threaten recovery if they are unprepared to deal with these. Although they may think of these mainly in relation to their addiction, this concept can also be applied to recovery from psychiatric illness.
2. In relation to addiction, high-risk people, places, events, and things are referred to as "triggers" because they precipitate cravings or increase vulnerability to using substances.
3. In relation to psychiatric illness, high-risk people and experiences can contribute to a recurrence. For example, the stress of living in a family in which hostility is expressed or the client is not supported can contribute to an episode of illness.
4. Emphasize that it is the client's use of active coping skills that ultimately determines the impact of people, places, events, and things.
5. Ask clients for specific examples and add to their list to cover a broad range of high-risk people, places, events, and things that can affect their recovery from addiction, psychiatric illness, or both. Common examples include the following:

   - Associating with drug dealers, other active addicts, or others who use drugs or get high on alcohol, even if they are not addicted.
   - Living with a spouse or partner who gets high on alcohol or other drugs or has an addiction.
   - Maintaining a relationship with a significant other who is nonsupportive of recovery, critical, violent, or unable to have a mutual "give-and-take" relationship.
   - Spending time at places or events where alcohol or drugs flow freely (i.e., parties, bars, concerts).
   - Associating sex with getting high or being unable to have sex unless high on drugs or alcohol.
   - Other places and things that trigger desire to use substances include: music, drug paraphernalia, money, the sight or smell of other substances, positive thoughts of getting high, certain sexual partners.

6. Discuss strategies to manage high-risk people, places, events, and things such as:
   - Avoiding high-risk people, places, and things.
   - Preparing ahead of time to cope with an unavoidable high-risk situation.
   - Ending relationships that are abusive or emotionally damaging.
   - Minimizing time spent with family members or significant others who are critical or nonsupportive of recovery.
   - Requesting a partner with a substance use or psychiatric disorder who represents a risk to the client's recovery get involved in treatment.
   - Gaining interpersonal strength to deal with destructive relationships through ongoing involvement in counseling.
   - Maintaining awareness of high-risk people, places, events, and things and talking to a support person to discuss ideas about how to manage these.

Supporting Materials

Dennis C. Daley, *Dual Diagnosis Workbook: Recovery Strategies for Substance Use and Mental Health Disorders*, pp. 102–105. Independence, Missouri: Herald House/Independence Press, 2003.

Dennis C. Daley, *Relapse Prevention Workbook for Recovering Alcoholics and Drug Dependent Persons*, pp. 4–7, 3rd ed. Holmes Beach, Florida: Learning Publications, 2001.

Video: *Resisting Social Pressures to Use Chemicals*. Wilmette, Illinois: Gerald T. Rogers Productions; phone: 1-800-227-9100; Web site: *www.gtrvideos.com*.

Video: *Staying Sober, Keeping Straight*. Wilmette, Illinois: Gerald T. Rogers Productions; phone: 1-800-227-9100; Web site: *www.gtrvideo.com*.

PE Group Topic #21
Managing Persistent Psychiatric Symptoms

Objectives

1. Define "persistent" or "chronic" symptoms of psychiatric illness.
2. Review strategies for clients to monitor their persistent or chronic symptoms to track significant changes over time.
3. Review strategies to manage persistent symptoms of psychiatric illness.

Points for Discussion

1. Many psychiatric disorders, especially those considered recurrent, persistent, or chronic, are "lifelong conditions." Clients may experience some symptoms more or less continuously. These are called "persistent" or "chronic" symptoms.

2. Ask clients for specific examples and add to their list as needed to generate a list of persistent mood, thinking, personality, or behavioral symptoms such as the following:

   - *Mood symptoms*: depression, emptiness, irritability, chronic anger, hypomania.
   - *Anxiety symptoms*: anxiety, fear or worry, obsessions, compulsions, panic symptoms, avoidance of situations causing anxiety.
   - *Psychotic symptoms*: hallucinations or delusions.
   - *Personality or behavioral symptoms*: impulsivity, self-destructive or suicidal behaviors, aggressiveness or angry outbursts, emptiness, obsessions, compulsions, avoidance, antisocial behavior.

3. Clients need to learn to live with persistent symptoms as these may never go totally away. The key is not whether or not a symptom is present but the severity of it and how it affects the client. For example, many clients have to live with some depression, anxiety, or hallucinations. However, once these symptoms worsen significantly, other interventions are needed.

4. Discuss the importance of completing a daily rating of persistent symptoms to monitor changes. When target symptoms go beyond their baseline or what clients can comfortably tolerate, different strategies need to be implemented.

5. Review the process of daily rating of persistent psychiatric symptoms.

   - The client identifies and labels persistent symptoms in his own words (e.g., hallucinations, voices, voices telling the client to do something bad).
   - Each persistent symptom is rated on a scale of one to ten, ten being the most severe and one being very mild.

6. Discuss when clients should ask for help from their counselor, doctor, or sponsor when their symptoms change significantly.

    - When they or others are concerned about suicidal or violent feelings.
    - When the level of personal suffering becomes high or intolerable.
    - When their symptoms interfere with their ability to take care of basic needs.
    - When they think they have done all they can do to fight off the symptom.

Supporting Materials

Robert Liberman, *Social and Independent Living Skills Symptom Management Module*, pp. 57–73. Los Angeles: UCLA Department of Psychiatry, 1988.

PE Group Topic #22
Managing Anger

Objectives

1. Define the three components of anger: feelings, thoughts, and behaviors.
2. Identify connections between anger and substance use or psychiatric disorders.
3. Review causes and effects of anger and the ways in which it is managed.
4. Review strategies to manage anger effectively in recovery.
5. Review strategies to cope with anger from other people.

Points for Discussion

1. Ask clients to define anger and discuss the degree to which it is a problem in their lives. Some will report chronic problems with anger and state they have a "short fuse." Others will state they have difficulty allowing themselves to feel angry or express it. Relate their answers to anger having these components:
   - Emotional (feelings)
   - Cognitive (thoughts and beliefs)
   - Behavioral (actions)
2. Discuss what clients learned from parents and others about anger and how to express it or deal with it in their relationships with others.
3. Review unhealthy and healthy ways of expressing anger:
   - *Unhealthy*: acting out and hurting others physically or verbally, hurting oneself, being passive and letting anger build up, drinking or using drugs, and acting in passive–aggressive ways.
   - *Healthy*: expressing it to others in a controlled manner when it is appropriate to do so, talking about feelings with a confidante, talking oneself out of being angry, engaging in activity that helps release or control anger, praying, or using anger as a motivator.
4. Ask clients to give examples of the effects of unhealthy anger management strategies on themselves and others.
   - *On self*: using substances, becoming enraged, depressed, or out of control.
   - *On others*: causing fear or worry, pushing others away emotionally, causing emotional damage in a relationship or causing it to end.
5. Discuss the connection between anger and methods of expression and substance use or psychiatric disorders.

- Anger can lead to substance use and be an excuse for relapse.
- Anger that controls a person can lead to acting out in ways that hurt others emotionally or physically.
- Anger that is not dealt with and suppressed can contribute to depression, self-harm, anxiety, low self-esteem, or internal turmoil.

6. Review strategies for managing anger and elicit examples from clients for each of the following categories.
    - *Verbal strategies*: talking about it directly with the person one is angry at, talking with a confidante to release feelings in a safe context, or getting support and another person's perspective.
    - *Cognitive or self-talk strategies*: changing thoughts, internal dialogue, or core beliefs, or using "slogans" of AA, NA, or DRA (e.g., "this too shall pass").
    - *Behavioral strategies*: going for a walk or exercising, redirecting one's activity, working around the house, praying or meditating, or going to an AA, NA, or DRA meeting to "drop off" anger.
    - *Medications*: when anger is intense, persistent, and acted on impulsively or aggressively, a mood stabilizer may be useful. An evaluation by a psychiatrist can determine if medications are needed.
7. Review a process to deal with angry feelings:
    - Step 1: Recognize anger in thoughts, feelings, and behaviors.
    - Step 2: Examine causes of anger.
    - Step 3: Evaluate the effects of anger and coping strategies used.
    - Step 4: Identify coping strategies to manage anger in each situation.
    - Step 5: Rehearse or practice new coping strategies.
    - Step 6: Put these into action, evaluate their effects, and change as needed.
8. Identify concerns of clients related to dealing with anger expressed by others.
9. Discuss strategies to cope with anger from other people.

Supporting Materials

Dennis C. Daley, *Dual Diagnosis Workbook: Recovery Strategies for Substance Use and Mental Health Disorders*, pp. 74–78. Independence, Missouri: Herald House/Independence Press, 2003.

Dennis C. Daley, *Managing Anger Workbook*, 2nd ed. Holmes Beach, Florida: Learning Publications, 2001.

Video: *Managing Anger in Recovery*. Wilmette, Illinois: Gerald T. Rogers Productions; phone: 1-800-227-9100; Web site: *www.gtrvideo.com*.

Video: *Why Are You So Angry?* Wilmette, Illinois: Gerald T. Rogers Productions, 1991. Phone: 1-800-227-9100; Web site: *www.gtrvideo.com*.

PE Group Topic #23
Managing Anxiety and Worry

Objectives

1. Define anxiety, worry, and anticipatory anxiety.
2. Review causes and effects of anxiety and worry.
3. Review anxiety and worry as symptoms common with anxiety disorders, depression, and substance use disorders.
4. Identify how substance use affects anxiety.
5. Review strategies for managing anxiety and worry.

Points for Discussion

1. Ask clients to define anxiety and worry and how the two go together.
   - Anxiety is the physical side and shows in symptoms such as nervous tension, tightness in stomach, and rapid heartbeat.
   - Worry is the psychological side and shows in thoughts and beliefs, which in turn affects behaviors.
2. Discuss "anticipatory" anxiety, which is the "fear" of something happening. Often anticipatory anxiety leads to "avoiding" the situation feared (e.g., a speech or a job interview).
3. Discuss causes of anxiety and worry and how these are common in many psychiatric and substance use disorders.
   - Anxiety is a symptom in generalized anxiety, obsessive–compulsive, panic, post-traumatic stress, and phobic disorders. These disorders are caused by multiple biological, psychological, and environmental factors.
   - Anxiety is a common symptom among people with mood, psychotic, and other psychiatric disorders.
   - Anxiety can be caused by substances or a symptom of withdrawal.
4. Review effects of anxiety on physical and emotional health and symptoms, relationships and substance use, particularly the use of benzodiazepines and alcohol.
5. Discuss treatment for anxiety disorders. Psychotherapy, medication, and combined treatments are used for anxiety disorders.
   - Cognitive, behavioral, and supportive therapies are used with anxiety disorders. Specialized therapies are used with disorders such as PTSD or phobias.

- The goals of therapy are to eliminate or reduce symptoms of the disorder, increase accurate thinking, improve functioning, and manage persistent symptoms of chronic disorders.
- Medication is used for moderate to severe types of anxiety disorders. The specific medicines used depend on the disorder, severity of symptoms, and impairment caused by the disorder.
- Selective serotonin reuptake inhibitors (SSRIs) are the most common medications used for panic disorder, phobias, obsessive–compulsive disorder, and post-traumatic stress disorder. Tricyclic antidepressants are used for panic disorder and PTSD, and monamine oxidase inhibitors are used for panic disorders.
- Nonaddictive anxiety agents such as BuSpar® and beta blockers are used for generalized anxiety disorders.
- Medications may be used to treat acute episodes of illness and to reduce the likelihood of future occurrences.
- Most of these medications take up to two weeks or longer to show the effects.

6. Review strategies for managing anxiety and worry. Emphasize the need for a variety of cognitive, affective, and behavioral strategies.
   - Identify and label anxiety and worry.
   - Find out what is causing anxiety and worry.
   - Get a physical examination.
   - Evaluate and change diet, especially the use of caffeine.
   - Evaluate lifestyle to identify sources of anxiety.
   - Change beliefs or thoughts that contribute to anxiety and worry.
   - Share anxious feelings and thoughts with others.
   - Learn to accept and live with persistent anxiety.
   - Set aside "worry" time each day.
   - Keep a written anxiety and worry journal.
   - Face the situations causing anxiety and worry. Do this gradually for situations that cause intense anxiety or fear.
   - Meditate and use relaxation techniques.
   - Practice proper breathing techniques.
   - Pray and ask for help from a Higher Power.

Supporting Materials

Dennis C. Daley, *Dual Diagnosis Workbook: Recovery Strategies for Substance Use and Mental Health Disorders*, pp. 79–83. Independence, Missouri: Herald House/Independence Press, 2003.

Daley and Salloum, *Understanding Major Anxiety Disorders and Addiction*, 2nd ed. Center City, Minnesota: Hazelden, 2003.

Video: *Recovering from Anxiety/Panic Disorder*. Wilmette, Illinois: Gerald T. Rogers Productions. Phone: 1-800-227-9100; Web site: *www.gtrvideo.com*, 1995.

Video: *Double Trouble: Recovery from Chemical Dependency and Mental Illness*. Part I—Mood and Anxiety. Wilmette, Illinois: Gerald T. Rogers Productions, 1990.

Video: *Understanding Major Anxiety Disorders and Addiction*. Center City, Minnesota: Hazelden, 1994.

PE Group Topic #24
Managing Boredom

Objectives

1. Identify ways that boredom impacts relapse.
2. Identify sources of boredom and "high-risk" times.
3. Review the importance of structure and routine in daily life.
4. Review strategies to manage boredom.

Points for Discussion

1. Ask clients to identify and discuss how boredom affects recovery from dual disorders. Problems associated with boredom include the following:
   - Relapse to alcohol or drug use.
   - Feeling depressed.
   - Getting involved in activities or relationships that may temporarily reduce boredom but create other problems.
2. Discuss how clients feel about living without alcohol, drugs, or partying.
3. Identify and list leisure activities given up due to the substance disorder.
4. Identify non-substance activities or situations that bring pleasure or are fun and that help reduce depression.
5. Identify and discuss the benefits of having structure in daily life.
   - Reduces the chances of engaging in high-risk situations that cause relapse.
   - Gives a sense of direction and purpose.
   - Forces clients to focus on goals and methods to achieve these goals.
6. Review practical coping strategies to reduce boredom.
   - Recognize boredom, high-risk times for it, and reasons for boredom.
   - Regain "lost" activities that are not substance-related.
   - Develop new leisure interests or hobbies.
   - Learn to appreciate the simple pleasures in life.
   - Build fun into day-to-day life.
   - Change thoughts and beliefs about boredom.
   - Evaluate relationship or job boredom before making major life changes.

- Deal with persistent feelings of boredom.
- Participate in support groups or recovery clubs.

7. *Option*: have clients complete a daily or weekly activities schedule to get them to practice building structure in their lives.
8. *Option*: discuss the issue of "emptiness" and "joylessness" associated with giving up substances, and how this contributes to both boredom and an inability to experience pleasure in normal activities.

Supporting Materials

Dennis C. Daley, *Dual Diagnosis Workbook: Recovery Strategies for Substance Use and Mental Health Disorders*, pp. 84–87. Independence, Missouri: Herald House/Independence Press, 2003.

Dennis C. Daley, *Relapse Prevention Workbook for Recovering Alcoholics and Drug Dependent Persons*, pp. 18–19.

Video: *Managing Feelings of Boredom and Emptiness*. Wilmette, Illinois: Gerald T. Rogers Production, 1994. Phone: 1-800-227-9100; Web site: *www.gtrvideo.com*.

PE Group Topic #25
Managing Depression

Objectives

1. Review types and symptoms of clinical depression.
2. Review causes and effects of depression.
3. Identify the relationships between substance use and depression.
4. Identify treatments for depression.
5. Review strategies to manage depression and improve mood.

Points for Discussion

1. Depression affects between 10 and 20 percent of adults and is twice as common among women than men. It is one of the leading causes of disability in the world and one of the leading causes of suicide.
2. About half who become depressed will experience a second episode at some time during their lives. For many people, depression is a chronic or recurrent condition.
3. Depression is very common among those with a substance use disorder. Untreated it can cause personal suffering, complicate recovery, and contribute to relapse.
4. Review types of depressive illness.
    - Major depression (single episode or recurrent with or without psychotic symptoms).
    - Seasonal depression.
    - Dysthymia (chronic, low-grade depression).
    - Bipolar depression.
    - Depression caused by substances or a medical condition.
5. Clinical depression is characterized by multiple symptoms that are persistent and last several weeks or longer. Functioning is often impaired as a result. Discuss "sub-syndromal depression" (having some symptoms of the disorder but not enough to meet full criteria).
6. Review symptoms of depression.
    - Feeling depressed, sad, irritable, or empty.
    - Feeling helpless, hopeless, or worthless.
    - Trouble experiencing pleasure or loss of interest in life.

- Significant gain or loss of weight without trying, loss of appetite.
- Falling asleep, waking up early, disrupted sleep, or sleeping too much.
- Feeling agitated or slowed down.
- Difficulty concentrating or remembering things.
- Loss or decrease in sexual desire.
- Thoughts of suicide, making a plan, or making an actual attempt.

7. Have clients identify factors that contributed to their depression. Use this to discuss biopsychosocial factors involved in depressive illness.
    - *Biological*: genetic vulnerability (it runs in families), or dysregulation of neurotransmitters in the brain.
    - *Psychological*: beliefs, personality, and coping skills deficits.
    - *Environmental*: family, job, economic, or other social problems.
    - *Interpersonal*: social skills deficits or unhealthy relationships.

8. Have clients give examples of how substance use affects depression. Both acute and chronic effects of drugs or withdrawal states cause symptoms of depression.

9. Have clients give examples of how depressed mood affects their substance use.

10. Ask clients how substance use can affect their recovery from depressive illness. Discuss how substance use can do the following:
    - Mask depressive symptoms.
    - Increase depressive symptoms.
    - Decrease motivation to recover.
    - Interfere with ability to make changes in self, lifestyle, or coping mechanisms.

11. Elicit examples of how alcohol and drug use affect psychiatric medications.
    - Substances can raise or lower the level of medications in the blood.
    - Substances may have a negative interaction with medications.
    - Substance use can also lower motivation to comply with medications.

12. Discuss treatment for depression. Psychotherapy, medication, electroshock therapy, and combined treatments are used for depressive illness.

13. There are many effective therapies for depression. The most common ones are cognitive–behavioral (CBT) and interpersonal psychotherapy (IPT). Both CBT and IPT may be used alone or in combination with medications.
    - The goals of therapy are to decrease or eliminate depressive symptoms, decrease inaccurate thinking or cognitive distortions, improve interpersonal effectiveness, deal with role transitions, reduce suicidal risk, and improve functioning.

- In cases of chronic depression, an additional goal is learning to manage persistent symptoms that do not totally remit.

14. Medication is used for moderate to severe types of depression. There are different types of antidepressants: selective serotonin reuptake inhibitors or (SSRIs), tricyclics (TCAs), and monamine oxidase inhibitors (MAOs). SSRIs are the most commonly used because they have less severe side effects. MAOs require a special diet.

    - For single episodes of depression, medications should be used for four to six months or longer after the episode remits. Otherwise, symptoms may return.
    - For recurrent episodes of depression, medications should be used continuously to reduce the likelihood of a future reoccurrence.
    - Most antidepressants take up to two weeks or longer to show the effects. Some people need more than one antidepressant for maximum benefit.

15. Discuss strategies to manage depression such as the following:

    - *Cognitive*: find out the problems that are contributing to depression and do something about them, change thoughts and beliefs contributing to depression or related symptoms, focus on positive experiences or successes.
    - *Interpersonal*: make amends, deal with loss or grief issues, deal with relationship problems or conflicts, participate in support groups.
    - *Emotional*: talk about feelings and problems with others, identify other emotions that may contribute to depression (i.e., guilt, anger, emptiness).
    - *Behavioral*: keep active and participate in pleasant activities, keep a journal or log of feelings, identify and plan social activities.
    - *Health and lifestyle*: get exercise, meditate, take medications as prescribed, do not stop taking medications without discussing this with a prescribing physician and/or counselor.

Supporting Materials

Dennis C. Daley, *Dual Diagnosis Workbook: Recovery Strategies for Substance Use and Mental Health Disorders*, pp 88–93. Independence, Missouri: Herald House/Independence Press, 2003.

Dennis C. Daley and Haskett, *Understanding Bipolar Illness and Addiction*, 2nd ed. Center City, Minnesota: Hazelden, 2003.

Dennis C. Daley and Michael E. Thase, *Understanding Depression and Addiction*, 2nd ed. Center City, Minnesota: Hazelden, 2003.

Video: *Double Trouble: Recovery from Chemical Dependency and Mental Illness.* Part I —Mood and Anxiety. Wilmette, Illinois: Gerald T. Rogers Productions, 1990. Phone 1-800-227-9100; Web site: *www.gtrvideo.com*.

Video: *Understanding Depression and Addiction*. Center City, Minnesota: Hazelden, 1994.

PE Group Topic #26
Managing Guilt and Shame

Objectives

1. Define "guilt" and "shame" and relate these feelings to dual disorders.
2. Encourage clients to share feelings of guilt and shame and specific experiences for which they feel guilty.
3. Review strategies to manage guilt and shame.
4. Discuss the importance of "changing behaviors" and "making amends" if feelings of guilt and shame are to be worked through.

Points for Discussion

1. Guilt and shame are common feelings among people with psychiatric, substance use, or dual disorders.
2. Have clients share their definitions of guilt and shame. Then discuss the following definitions:
   - Guilt refers to feeling bad about behaviors (actions or inactions).
   - Shame refers to feeling bad about oneself ("I'm defective," "I'm weak," "I'm a failure," "I'm less than").
3. Elicit examples of specific behaviors for which clients feel guilty such as the following:
   - Failure to be responsible as a parent, spouse, or adult child.
   - Not participating in family activities or failure to acknowledge occasions such as birthdays, graduations, anniversaries, holidays, or other events.
   - Not fulfilling obligations at work, home, or in the community.
   - Taking advantage of, lying to, or conning others.
   - Committing crimes.
   - Hurting others verbally, physically, or emotionally.
   - Spending family income on substances.
   - Failure to support one's family.
4. Encourage clients to talk about what it feels like to have dual disorders and some of the things they have done or failed to do that contribute to their guilt.
5. Reframe "shame" and talk about addiction and psychiatric disorders as "no-fault illnesses." Emphasize that people do not purposely set out to acquire any of these illnesses. However, it is important that clients accept responsibility to recover.

6. Discuss coping strategies for working through guilt and shame.
   - Recognize and accept feelings of guilt and shame.
   - Take time to work through guilt and shame. There are no quick fixes for working through these feelings.
   - Accept dual disorders as "no-fault" illnesses.
   - Share feelings of guilt and shame with others in recovery, a counselor, or religious person.
   - Use the Twelve Step program of AA, NA, or DRA.
   - Make amends to others hurt by the dual disorders.
   - Seek forgiveness from others.
   - Pray to and seek help from a Higher Power.

Supporting Materials

Dennis C. Daley, *Coping with Feelings Workbook*, pp. 51–56. 2nd ed. Holmes Beach, Florida: Learning Publications, 2003.

Twelve Step handouts.

PE Group Topic #27
Sharing Positive Feelings in Recovery

Objectives

1. Discuss the importance of expressing positive feelings toward others.
2. Identify positive feelings.
3. Identify strategies for sharing positive feelings and potential benefits to relationships of sharing feelings.

Points for Discussion

1. An important component of emotional competence is being able to experience and express positive emotions or feelings toward others.

2. Ask group members to share positive feelings that they have experienced and that they believe are important. Add to their examples as needed and cover a range of examples such as the following:
   - Love and affection
   - Hopefulness
   - Joy
   - Caring
   - Glad, happy, thankful
   - Passionate
   - Playful

3. Although much discussion in recovery focuses on coping with negative feelings (anger, guilt, depression), it is also important to focus on positive feelings. Such feelings are a great source of satisfaction in relationships and necessary for relationships to deepen.

4. Similar to other feelings, positive feelings show in behaviors and what is said to others. Stress that saying positive things without backing these up with actions will have limited impact. For example:
   - A person can tell another "I love you" but treat them poorly. These words will have little impact as a result.
   - A person can tell another "I love you" and do nice things for this other person and show this love by their actions and their words.

5. Ask group members to share their thoughts on the importance of expressing positive feelings. Add to their ideas to include some of the following examples of benefits of sharing positive feelings:

- Helps build relationships and enhance connectedness to others.
- Helps balance out negative feelings in relationships.
- Contributes to satisfaction in life.
- Promotes better mental health.

6. Ask group members to identify ways positive feelings can be shared.
   - In words: elicit specific examples such as making caring or loving remarks, expressing love or empathy, and making a statement conveying appreciation of another person.
   - In actions: elicit specific examples such as taking care of another person; doing something nice for them; surprising them with a card, letter or gift; or helping them in time of need.

Supporting Materials

Dennis C. Daley, *Coping with Feelings Workbook*, pp. 63–65. 2nd ed. Holmes Beach, Florida: Learning Publications, 2003.

PE Group Topic #28
Dual Disorders and the Family

Objectives

1. Review psychiatric and substance use disorders as familial disorders, and discuss the impact of these disorders on the family unit and its members.
2. Review concerns and questions of families related to dual disorders.
3. Review the importance of involving the family in treatment and recovery.
4. Identify situations in which a family member may need help with her own substance use or psychiatric disorder.
5. Review recovery strategies for family members.

Points for Discussion

1. Psychiatric and substance use disorders run in families. Prevalence rates are significantly higher among first-degree relatives (children and siblings) of an affected person than the general population.
2. Psychiatric and substance use disorders are associated with many family problems. The family unit and individual members are affected, sometimes in profound ways.
3. Effects of dual disorders on the family vary from mild to serious. The actual effects depend on the severity of the disorders, behaviors of the dual disordered member, and coping skills and support systems of family members.
4. Ask clients for examples of how their family unit and individual members were affected by their disorders. Expand on their list to include problems related to the following:
   - Family mood and atmosphere.
   - Communication and interaction in the family.
   - Psychological and emotional effects on family members (e.g., anger, depression, confusion, anxiety, frustration, guilt, and shame).
   - Financial effects.
   - Family breakup due to divorce, separation, incarceration, or having children taken by child welfare services.
5. Discuss family recovery issues for the dual disordered member.
   - Acknowledging the impact of disorders on the family.
   - Encouraging family involvement in treatment and recovery.
   - Making amends to family members hurt by these disorders.

- Taking an active role in the lives of family members.
6. Discuss the importance of family involvement in assessment and treatment. There are a variety of types of sessions the family may attend (evaluation, education, counseling). Family involvement can help in two general ways:
    - Supporting the dual diagnosed member's recovery.
    - Gaining help and support for the family and its members.
7. Discuss the possibility that other family members, including children, may have psychiatric or substance use disorders requiring treatment.
8. Discuss "red flags" for determining if a family member needs help. An evaluation should be sought when the family member has the following:
    - Symptoms of an anxiety, mood, psychotic, personality, eating, or impulse control disorder (e.g., depression, mood swings, or suicidality).
    - Threats of violence or suicide or actual behaviors harmful to self or others.
    - Evidence of a substance abuse or dependence disorder.
    - Impairment in functioning at home, school, or work caused by a psychiatric and/or substance use disorder.
    - Personal distress or suffering resulting from psychiatric symptoms or a substance use disorder.
9. Family members benefit from counseling and participation in support groups such as Al-Anon, Nar-Anon, and NAMI (National Alliance of the Mentally Ill). These help reduce the family burden and enable family members to become educated about dual disorders and learn coping skills.
10. Discuss recovery strategies for families and their members.
    - Acknowledging and accepting the dual disorders and the impact on everyone in the family.
    - Accepting the need for help and support for family members, not just the impaired dual disordered member. Help may come from professionals, other members of mutual support groups, or both.
    - Reducing behaviors that "enable" the affected family member.
    - Learning to "detach" and set limits, but in a kind supportive manner.
    - Developing realistic expectations of the impaired family member and acknowledging success, even when it occurs in small steps.
    - Developing a plan for psychiatric emergencies (suicidal threats or gestures, violence, poor treatment adherence, or relapse of either disorder).
    - Focusing on self (feelings, goals, dreams, and desired changes) not just the impaired family member.
    - Helping children in the family understand and deal with the impact of the disorders on them.

Supporting Materials

Dennis C. Daley, *Dual Diagnosis Workbook: Recovery Strategies for Substance Use and Mental Health Disorders*, pp 96–101. Independence, Missouri: Herald House/Independence Press, 2003.

Dennis C. Daley and J. Sinberg-Spear, *A Family Guide to Coping with Dual Disorders*, 3rd ed. Center City, Minnesota: Hazelden, 2003.

D. Marsh and R. Dickens, *How to Cope with Mental Illness in Your Family*. New York: J.P. Tarcher, 1998.

Video: *Psychiatric Illness and the Family*. Wilmette, Illinois: Gerald T. Rogers Production, 1995. Phone: 1-800-227-9100; Web site: *www.gtrvideo.com*.

Video: *Together: Families in Recovery*. Wilmette, Illinois: Gerald T. Rogers Productions. Phone: 1-800-227-9100; Web site: *www.gtrvideo.com*.

PE Group Topic #29
Impact of Disorders on Children

Objectives

1. Review effects of psychiatric, substance use, and dual disorders on children.
2. Identify ways that parents can help their children.
3. Recognize that some children may need professional help.

Points for Discussion

1. Psychiatric, substance use, and dual disorders effect children in many ways.
2. Studies of children of parents with a substance use disorder (SUD) show that, compared to children who do not have a parent with an SUD, these kids have higher rates of the following:
   - Alcohol or drug abuse.
   - Mood and anxiety disorders.
   - Oppositional disorders, delinquency, aggression, and conduct disturbances.
   - Impulsivity, inattention, and irritability.
   - Academic problems (poorer performance in school and lower scores on IQ tests).
3. Many of these children worry about their parents, feel unwanted, angry, anxious, or hopeless, act in defiant ways, or feel that a parent's substance abuse hurts relationships within and outside of the family.
4. Studies of children of parents with a psychiatric disorder show that these children are more prone to developing a psychiatric disorder. These kids also feel an emotional burden similar to children in families with a parent who has an SUD.
5. Even adult children can feel the adverse effects from a parent's psychiatric illness, SUD, or dual disorders.
6. Parents and adults can help children who have been exposed to a family member's psychiatric, substance use, or dual disorders by the following:
   - Educating the children about dual disorders.
   - Encouraging children to ask questions and talk about their feelings and experiences related to a parent's disorders.
   - Accepting that children often feel an emotional burden due to a parent's illness, regardless of the type of illness.

- Protecting the child from violence, intoxication, and other high-risk behaviors.
- Providing the child with hope that things can get better in the family.
- Sharing activities with the child.
- Taking an interest in the child's activities and relationships.
- Focusing on the child's strengths and building resiliencies.
- Getting the child to attend treatment sessions with the parent(s).
- Getting help for any child who shows serious academic, substance abuse, or psychiatric problems (anxiety, depression, suicidality, violence, problems at school, or with the law).

Supporting Materials

Dennis C. Daley, *Dual Diagnosis Workbook: Recovery Strategies for Substance Use and Mental Health Disorders*, pp. 100–101. Independence, Missouri: Herald House/Independence Press, 2003.

Dennis C. Daley and J. Sinberg-Spear, *I Can Talk about What Hurts: A Book for Kids in Homes Where There's Chemical Dependency*. Center City, Minnesota: Hazelden, 1993.

Video: *Reflections from the Heart of a Child*. Center City, Minnesota: Hazelden. Phone: 1-800-257-7810; Fax: 651-213-4411; Web site: *www.hazelden.org*.

PE Group Topic #30
Impact of Dual Disorders on Relationships

Objectives

1. Identify effects of dual disorders on relationships.
2. Identify ways to begin repairing some of the damage done to relationships.
3. Review strategies to improve communication and relationships.

Points for Discussion

1. Relationships with family and others are often hurt by behaviors associated with substance use, psychiatric illness, or both. These effects range from mild to severe.

2. Ask clients to provide examples of behaviors and adverse effects of their disorders on people in their lives. Add to this list to provide a broad overview of various behaviors and adverse interpersonal effects of dual disorders such as the following:

   - Broken or lost relationships.
   - Distrust from others.
   - Lying, stealing, or conning others, especially in relation to getting or using substances or covering-up use.
   - Emotional upset (anger, disappointment, confusion, anxiety or worry, depression).
   - An inability to take care of responsibilities toward others (e.g., can't fulfill parental role, relate on mutual level with partner, provide for family).
   - Emotional or physical violence toward others.

3. An important aspect of recovery is repairing the damage caused in relationships. Ask clients to give examples of strategies they can use to begin improving relationships damaged by their disorders. Add additional ideas as needed to their list and cover the following strategies:

   - Acknowledging that others were affected by the dual disorders.
   - Providing information regarding dual disorders and recovery to family or significant others.
   - Inviting family or significant others to treatment sessions.
   - Encouraging family or significant others to attend self-help groups.
   - Openly discussing the impact of dual disorders on the family or significant others, allowing others to share what it was like for them.
   - Working Steps 8 and 9 of the Twelve Step program (making amends steps).

4. Discuss strategies to improve communication and relationships. Some examples include:
   - Listen to the concerns, problems, and needs of others.
   - Show empathy and compassion toward others.
   - Provide emotional support to others.
   - Do things to help others.
   - Express positive feelings toward others.
   - Be respectful when discussing problems or conflicts with others.
   - Do not allow negative feelings to dictate how you act toward others.
   - Share mutual interests with others.
   - Maintain an active social life.
5. Verbal strategies to improve relationships will have little or no impact if they are not backed up by positive behavior change. For example, it does little good to apologize for verbal or physical aggression if the client does not change these behaviors.

Supporting Materials

Dennis C. Daley, *Double Recovery: Managing Your Substance Use and Mental Health Disorders*. Memphis, Tennessee: Foundations, 2004.

Dennis C. Daley, *Improving Communication and Relationships*. Holmes Beach, Florida: Learning Publications, 1996.

Terence T. Gorski, *Getting Love Right*. New York, New York: Fireside/Parkside, 1993.

Video: *Coping with Family and Interpersonal Conflicts*. Wilmette, Illinois: Gerald T. Rogers Productions. Phone: 1-800-227-9100; Web site: *www.gtrvideo.com*.

PE Group Topic #31
Saying No to Getting High

Objectives

1. Teach clients to anticipate direct and indirect social pressures to use substances.
2. Identify the effects of social pressures on thoughts, feelings, and behaviors.
3. Teach clients about "relapse set-ups"—how they put themselves in high risk social pressure situations (consciously or unconsciously).
4. Review strategies to refuse social pressures to use alcohol or other drugs.

Points for Discussion

1. Social pressure to use substances is one of the most common relapse risk factors with substance disorders. It is not the social pressure itself, but client's ability to manage it that determines if a relapse occurs.
2. Ask clients to provide examples of direct and indirect social pressures they have faced or expect to face in the future. These will fall in one of these categories:
    - *People*: family members or friends who use, people with whom clients drank or got high, and drug dealers.
    - *Places*: bars, parties, or other places where substances were used.
    - *Events or situations*: weddings, graduations, holiday celebrations, sporting events, concerts, or family events.
3. Set up role plays where a client is offered alcohol or drugs by another person. Ask other group members observing the role play to identify with the client being offered substances and to pay attention to their thoughts and feelings.
4. After the role play, process it with the actors and other group members. Focus on the following questions:
    - What do clients feel when confronted by social pressures to use?
    - What thoughts come to their minds when offered alcohol or drugs?
    - How do social pressures impact motivation to stay sober?
    - What can they do to refuse offers of substances?
5. *Option*: have clients pair up in dyads. Each offers the other alcohol or drugs. After this experience, discuss the same questions listed above.
6. *Option*: in the role play, instruct the individual offering alcohol or drugs to add an offer of a "good time" or sex. A male client might feel more vulnerable to an offer by

a female to get high because of the association between sex and getting high with a woman (or vice versa). A variation is to use male-male or female-female scenarios in order to address social pressures experienced by gay men and lesbian women.

7. After the group processes the role play, review coping strategies.

- Avoidance of high-risk social pressure situations.
- Verbal (ways to say no).
- Behavioral (ways to reduce or deal with unavoidable social pressures).

8. Also, discuss the issue of "ambivalence," (i.e., this role play often helps clients realize that part of them still wants to get high, and they "miss the action").

Supporting Materials

Dennis C. Daley, *Dual Diagnosis Workbook: Recovery Strategies for Substance Use and Mental Health Disorders*, pp. 102–104. Independence, Missouri: Herald House/Independence Press, 2003.

Dennis C. Daley, *Relapse Prevention Workbook for Recovering Alcoholics and Drug Dependent Persons*, pp. 12–14. 3rd ed. Holmes Beach, Florida: Learning Publications, 2001.

Video: *Resisting Social Pressures to Use Chemical*. Wilmette, Illinois: Gerald T. Rogers Productions. Phone: 1-800-227-9100; Web site: *www.gtrvideo.com*.

Video: *Staying Sober, Keeping Straight*. Wilmette, Illinois: Gerald T. Rogers Productions. Phone: 1-800-227-9100; Web site: *www.gtrvideo.com*.

PE Group Topic #32
Resisting Pressures to Stop Taking Psychiatric Medications

Objectives

1. Teach clients to anticipate pressures to stop taking their psychiatric medications.
2. Identify effects of such pressures on their thoughts, feelings, and behaviors.
3. Identify strategies to handle pressures to stop taking psychiatric medications.

Points for Discussion

1. Family, friends, and members of mutual support groups may pressure people in recovery to stop taking psychiatric medications. This occurs due to erroneous beliefs about medication use among those with a substance use disorder.

2. Ask group members for examples of situations in which they were pressured to stop taking medications (or have some scenarios available to role play should clients be unable to provide examples) such as the following:
   - A member of AA, NA, or CA tells a client that she is not sober because she takes medications.
   - A family member or friend tells a client that she should not be on medication.
   - A member of a support group, family member, or friend tells the client of his own "bad experiences" with psychiatric medications and suggests the client might want to reconsider the need for medications.

3. Choose one or two of these situations and set up role plays where one client is told by another that he should stop taking medications. Use the role plays to demonstrate the issues related to pressures from others to stop taking medications.

4. Ask clients observing the role play to identify with the person being pressured to stop taking medicine and to pay close attention to what they think and feel.

5. After the role play, discuss the effects of such situations on the client's thoughts, feelings, and behaviors. Focus on factors involved in making a decision on taking medications or giving in to pressure from others to stop.

6. Ask clients to discuss the implications of stopping psychiatric medications. Reinforce the difference between drugs used to get high or drunk and those used to treat medical or psychiatric illnesses.

7. Review strategies to manage pressures to stop taking medications.
   - Informing a sponsor about being on psychiatric medications.

- Being discreet about who to tell about taking psychiatric medications.
- Telling the person pressuring the client that medicines are being used for a medical problem.
- Reminding the person pressuring the client that he may relapse to psychiatric illness or alcohol or drug use if medications are stopped.
- Asking the person if they would make the same request regarding medicines for a heart condition or diabetes.
- Keeping in mind that only a doctor should tell the client when they should stop taking medications.
- Leaving the situation if pressures become too great.

8. Option: have clients pair up in dyads. In each dyad, one client tells the other client that he should get off all drugs, including medications from "shrinks." Each client practices responding to this situation. Then the group as a whole discusses the experience, focusing on thoughts, feelings, and behaviors generated by such pressure. Both ineffective and positive coping strategies can be identified.

Supporting Materials

The AA Member, Medication and Other Drugs. AA World Services.

Index cards with examples of common scenarios in which a client is pressured to stop taking psychiatric medication.

PE Group Topic #33
Building a Recovery Network

Objectives

1. Review the importance of having a recovery network to support recovery.
2. Identify common resistances and problems in building a recovery network (e.g., guilt, shame, and embarrassment; inability to ask for help).
3. Assess current social networks of clients to determine changes needed to support their recovery.
4. Identify other potential sources of support (individuals and organizations).

Points for Discussion

1. Discuss the importance of a recovery network and working a "we" rather than an "I" program.
2. Review reasons why clients might not ask for help. Some examples include the following:
   - Feelings of guilt, shame, or embarrassment.
   - Fear that the other person being asked for help will refuse.
   - The client does not know what to say when asking for help from others.
   - The client does not know how to ask for support.
   - The client does not have a confidante or sober people to rely on.
3. Discuss why family members or other people may not be willing to help or support clients. Some examples include the following:
   - They may be upset or angry at the client for things that he did or failed to do.
   - They may have been cheated out of money or taken advantage of in other ways.
   - They may have serious problems themselves that interfere with their ability to show support or give help.
4. Ask clients to identify people and organizations to support their recovery. These may include the following:
   - Family members, friends, and coworkers.
   - AA, NA, or DRA members and groups.
   - Mental health support groups and group members.
   - Members of a treatment group.

- Church, religious organizations, other organizations, or community groups.
5. Ask clients to state specific ways others can help or support them such as the following:
    - Listening to their problems or difficulties.
    - Offering advice and help.
    - Spending time in an enjoyable activity together.
    - Discussing ways to use the "tools" of recovery (especially true for sponsors and other members of support groups).
    - Helping with a practical need (ride to a meeting, help moving furniture).
    - Pointing out early relapse warning signs that the client may ignore.
6. Discuss the importance of "making amends" to others (especially family members and close friends hurt by behaviors associated with either illness) before asking for help and support.
7. Review strategies for asking for help. Use role plays to illustrate the process of asking for help and to help clients become aware of how difficult this can be. Role plays can focus on concrete situations such as asking for a sponsor, asking someone to listen to a problem, or asking someone for a favor.
8. After conducting role plays, ask group members to discuss their thoughts and feelings about asking for help. State that some clients may have to practice asking for help before they will feel comfortable doing so.
9. Emphasize the need to work with others and to ask for help and support while still taking responsibility for recovery. Strongly emphasize the importance of AA, NA, DRA, dual recovery groups, and mental health support groups.

Supporting Materials

Dennis C. Daley, *Dual Diagnosis Workbook: Recovery Strategies for Substance Use and Mental Health Disorders*, pp. 105–106. Independence, Missouri: Herald House/Independence Press, 2003.

Dennis C. Daley, *Improving Communication and Relationships*, pp. 29–41. Holmes Beach, Florida: Learning Publications, 1996.

Video: *Building a Recovery Network and Sponsorship*. Wilmette, Illinois: Gerald T. Rogers Productions, 1999. Phone: 1-800-227-9100; Web site: *www.gtrvideo.com*.

PE Group Topic #34
Self-Help Programs

Objectives

1. Review the importance of self-help programs in recovery.
2. Provide information on types of self-help programs for substance use, psychiatric, and dual disorders.
3. Provide information on the "tools" of self-help programs (meetings, slogans, literature).
4. Identify ways a "sponsor" can aid recovery.
5. Stress the helpfulness of "recovery clubs."

Points for Discussion

1. Ask clients about their experiences in self-help groups—types of groups attended, ways groups have been helpful, and resistances to attending groups.
2. Discuss resistances to attending self-help groups and ways to overcome these resistances such as the following:
   - Attending different groups.
   - Attending at least twelve meetings before judging groups.
   - Closely examining the reasons for resistance to support groups.
   - Getting help and support in facing fears of talking in groups and sharing personal information.
3. Review the types of self-help groups for clients with dual disorders.
   - AA, NA, CA, Rational Recovery, SMART Recovery, and Women for Sobriety for substance use disorders.
   - Emotions Anonymous, Recovery Inc., and other specific disorder based support groups (i.e., depression and manic-depressive support groups) for psychiatric disorders.
   - Double Trouble, MISA, and DRA for dual disorders.
4. Discuss how self-help groups aid recovery.
   - Providing information.
   - Getting help and support from others who have similar problems.
   - Getting exposure to the Twelve Step program.
   - Having an opportunity to work with a sponsor.

- Helping structure free time by involvement in recovery oriented activities.
- Learning skills to manage the dual disorders.

5. Review the role of a "sponsor" and how to get one in AA, NA, or DRA.
   - Mentors the group member (teaches the ropes).
   - Provides support.
   - Helps work the Twelve Steps.
   - Serves as a model for success.
6. Review the different types and formats of self-help meetings:
   - Open discussion of recovery issues raised by participants.
   - Discussions on Twelve Steps of AAA/NA, or a reading from the "Big Book" of AA or "Basic Text" of NA.
   - Lead meetings where a personal story of illness and recovery is shared.
   - Guest speakers for special events.
   - Special meetings for specific disorders; gender specific; groups for gays or lesbians, health care professionals, business people, students.
7. Discuss the Twelve Step program and how this can be used in ongoing recovery to address the challenges of recovery (i.e., acceptance of addiction, relying on a Higher Power, identifying character defects, taking a daily inventory, making amends).
8. Review the other "tools of recovery."
   - Slogans
   - Literature
   - Use of a Higher Power
   - Serenity Prayer
9. Emphasize that recovery is a "we" rather than an "I" endeavor, and much support is available for any person willing to use this support.
10. Discuss the purpose of "recovery clubs" and provide information on local clubs.

Supporting Materials

Dennis C. Daley, *Dual Diagnosis Workbook: Recovery Strategies for Substance Use and Mental Health Disorders*, pp. 107–112. Independence, Missouri: Herald House/Independence Press, 2003.

Copy of the Serenity Prayer, slogans, Twelve Steps of Recovery of AA/NA, or modified Steps for DRA or Double Trouble Groups, and/or local meeting lists.

Video: *Compliance with Medications and Self-Help Programs*, 1999. Wilmette, Illinois: Gerald T. Rogers Productions. Phone: 1-800-227-9100; Web site: *www.gtrvideo.com*.

PE Group Topic #35
Changing Negative or Inaccurate Thinking

Objectives
1. Review the impact of beliefs and thoughts on feelings, behaviors, psychiatric symptoms, and substance use.
2. Identify "cognitive distortions" that impact on relapse of either disorder.
3. Identify strategies to change cognitive distortions or inaccurate thinking.
4. Introduce the concept of "stinking thinking" of AA, NA, or DRA programs.

Points for Discussion
1. Elicit examples of inaccurate, distorted, negative, or "stinking thinking." Ask how thinking impacts client's feelings and behaviors.
    - Thinking can contribute to psychiatric symptoms, such as anxiety or depression.
    - Thinking can lead to substance use.
    - Thinking can affect satisfaction in life.
2. Provide examples of cognitive distortions or inaccurate thinking such as the following:
    - Black-and-white thinking or viewing situations in extremes, without accepting that there are "gray" in-between areas.
    - Making things worse than they are.
    - Making generalizations based on a single experience.
    - Expecting the worst to happen or expecting to fail.
    - Ignoring the positive and focusing only on the negative.
    - Jumping to conclusions without all the facts.
3. Strategies to change thoughts and beliefs include the following:
    - Be aware of thinking patterns.
    - Check the evidence for negative or inaccurate thoughts.
    - Challenge cognitive distortions or stinking thinking.
    - Focus less on the negative and more on the positive.
    - Keep a journal to recall and dispute inaccurate thoughts.
    - Regularly review benefits of recovery, progress, and appreciate efforts to change.

- Learn and use the slogans in AA or NA.
- Read materials written about how to improve thinking.

4. Review a process for challenging cognitive distortions and negative thinking.
   - Step 1: identify the belief or thought.
   - Step 2: state what is faulty or incorrect about it.
   - Step 3: identify two to four counterstatements for each belief or thought.

5. Have clients identify specific examples of their thinking to practice using these three steps. Ask clients to share their examples. Other clients can add more ideas and counterstatements for the examples shared.

6. Discuss the importance of small changes. For example, if a client can reduce negative thinking by 10 percent, this is good progress. Clients should not expect major changes to occur quickly. Cognitive changes require practice.

7. Encourage clients to continue their work by practicing changing thoughts and beliefs between group sessions.

Supporting Materials

David Burns, *Ten Days to Self Esteem*. New York: Quill, 1993.

Dennis C. Daley, *Dual Diagnosis Workbook: Recovery Strategies for Substance Use and Mental Health Disorders*, pp. 123–126. Independence, Missouri: Herald House/Independence Press, 2003.

Dennis C. Daley, *Overcoming Negative Thinking*. Center City, Minnesota: Hazelden, 1988.

PE Group Topic #36
Changing Self-Defeating Behaviors

Objectives

1. Review self-defeating behaviors associated with dual disorders.
2. Review self-destructive behaviors associated with dual disorders.
3. Help clients identify their own self-defeating and self-destructive behaviors.
4. Review strategies to change these behaviors.

Points for Discussion

1. Define self-defeating behaviors as those that threaten the client's physical health, emotional well-being, relationships, financial status, ability to get or keep a job, or ability to function in other areas of life.
2. Elicit examples of self-defeating behaviors from clients. Mention some of the following to provide concrete examples:
   - Jumping from one relationship to the next.
   - Getting easily bored with a partner.
   - Moving in with a partner after knowing this person for a short period of time.
   - Picking up strangers and having sex with them.
   - Getting involved too quickly in a romantic relationship.
   - Getting involved in relationships that are physically or emotionally abusive.
   - Using intimidation and anger to keep people on their guard.
   - Quitting jobs impulsively or underperforming at work.
   - Managing money poorly and getting deep in debt.
   - Gambling too much or compulsively.
   - Compulsive sexual behavior.
   - Getting involved in illegal activities or criminal behaviors.
3. Define self-destructive behaviors as those that cause physical or psychological harm to the client or another person. Examples include the following:
   - Suicidal threats or acts.
   - Acts such as cutting or burning oneself or punching a wall.
   - Physical violence toward other people or threats of violence.

- Breaking or destroying property.
- Overdosing on drugs or alcohol.
- Any compulsive behaviors (gambling, sex, spending).

4. Personality disorders and bipolar disorder often involve impulsive behaviors that are self-destructive or self-defeating.

5. Some self-destructive or self-defeating behaviors caused by poor judgment during an episode of illness such as a mania or a psychotic break may stop when the psychiatric illness is stabilized.

6. Changing these behaviors involves gaining an awareness of what they are and what causes them. This puts clients in a better position to devise action plans to reduce or stop them.

7. Have clients identify one self-defeating or self-destructive behavior they want to change. Discuss ways they can change this behavior.

8. Summarize strategies that may be used to change these behaviors. Use some of the examples of coping strategies given by group members.

    - Changing the way a person thinks about himself, other people, and the world; accepting responsibility for problems; and making a commitment to change.
    - Completing an inventory of strengths and deficits or character defects. Working Steps 4 and 10 of the AA/NA/DRA program with a sponsor is an excellent way to identify and change personality problems.
    - Decreasing or stopping behaviors that cause problems such as violence toward others, impulsive acting out, or controlling impulsive behaviors associated with personality problems.
    - Increasing behaviors that are prosocial or helpful toward others.
    - Increasing personal control over emotions and how these are expressed.
    - Some professional treatments, such as cognitive therapy, help clients change thoughts, underlying beliefs, and their related behaviors.
    - Personality disorders that involve behaviors as acting violently toward others or hurting oneself often respond to mood stabilizing medications. An evaluation by a psychiatrist can determine if medicines can help a client.

Supporting Materials

Dennis C. Daley, *Dual Diagnosis Workbook: Recovery Strategies for Substance Use and Mental Health Disorders*, pp. 114–117. Independence, Missouri: Herald House/Independence Press, 2003.

Dennis C. Daley and R.D. Weiss, *Understanding Personality Problems and Addiction.* 2nd ed. Center City, Minnesota: Hazelden, 2003.

Video: *Understanding Suicide and Addiction,* 2003. Center City, Minnesota: Hazelden. Web site: *www.hazelden.org*.

PE Group Topic #37
Changing Personality Problems

Objectives

1. Define personality and personality problems.
2. Review the connection between personality problems and addiction.
3. Identify problematic traits that may hinder client's recovery or well-being.
4. Review strategies to change one problematic personality trait identified.

Points for Discussion

1. Ask clients to define personality and give examples. Then, define personality as a person's characteristic way of seeing the world and relating to other people. It shows in behaviors and patterns of relating to self and to other people.

2. Personality problems are common among people with substance use and psychiatric disorders. There are a couple of ways of looking at this.

    - Personality traits can cause problems but not be part of a personality disorder.

    - Personality disorders are long-term conditions in which certain ingrained traits cause significant problems in living or personal distress.

    - The more common personality disorders among those with substance use disorders include borderline and antisocial disorders.

3. Elicit examples of personality problems, and ask clients to talk about ways these have influenced drug and alcohol use, caused problems in their relationship with other people, or caused personal distress.

4. Ask clients if they have heard the term "character defect" used in Twelve Step programs. Ask them to define how they relate to it in terms of their own personality. Relate this concept to changing problematic personality traits as part of ongoing recovery.

5. Discuss the importance of viewing personality traits on a continuum and that even some that are identified as negative or problematic may have positive aspects to them. Traits identified as positive can have negative aspects to them.

    - For example, aggressiveness can get one into trouble if it is used to hurt other people or to put other people down. However, aggressiveness can be helpful in business situations, athletic situations, or situations where other people want to take advantage of the client.

    - Similarly, kindness can be a positive trait and help one develop solid reciprocal relationships. However, if one is too kind and always "giving to others," then they may harbor resentment on the inside or feel dissatisfied in their relationships.

- Therefore it is usually not the trait in and of itself but the degree that it affects the person in recovery that is important.

6. Have clients identify one trait they would like to change and discuss ways they can change. Use these examples to point out how people change personality problems over time. Emphasize that change requires practice.

    - Change beliefs about the trait and associated behavior. For example, a client who is too passive and unable to express anger can work on changing the belief that "anger is bad and should be avoided at all costs" into "anger is a normal part of life."

    - Change behavior associated with the trait. For example, a passive client can practice being assertive and expressing ideas, thoughts, and feelings rather than holding these in.

    - The strategies reviewed in the previous section on changing self-defeating and self-destructive behaviors are also relevant to personality disorders.

Supporting Materials

Dennis C. Daley, *Dual Diagnosis Workbook: Recovery Strategies for Substance Use and Mental Health Disorders*, pp. 118–122. Independence, Missouri: Herald House/Independence Press 2003.

Dennis C. Daley and R.D. Weiss, *Understanding Personality Problems and Addiction*, 2nd ed. Center City, Minnesota: Hazelden, 2003.

Video: *Recovering from Borderline Personality Disorder*. Wilmette, Illinois: Gerald T. Rogers Productions, 1995. Phone: 1-800-227-9100; Web site: *www.gtrvideo.com*.

Video: *Double Trouble: Recovery from Chemical Dependency and Mental Illness*. Part II—Personality Disorders, Wilmette, Illinois: Gerald T. Rogers Productions, 1990. Phone: 1-800-227-9100; Web site: *www.gtrvideo.com*.

Video: *Understanding Personality Problems and Addiction*. Center City, Minnesota: Hazelden. Phone: 1-800-257-7810; Web site: *www. hazelden.org*.

PE Group Topic #38
Developing Spirituality

Objectives

1. Review spirituality as a domain of recovery.
2. Identify ways that spirituality can aid recovery and self-change.
3. Help client understand the "we" versus the "I" aspect of recovery.
4. Identify steps of the AA, NA, CA, or DRA program that address spirituality.

Points for Discussion

1. Recovery is multidimensional. One important aspect is spirituality. Ask clients to define spirituality and what it means to their recovery.
2. Discuss "values and meaning" as an aspect of spirituality. Ask clients to talk about which relationships, activities, or values give them the most meaning and purpose in their life.
3. Spiritual values include honesty, faith, hope, humility, courage, compassion, forgiveness, and altruism or service to others.
4. Spiritual activities include self-reflection, meditation, prayer, and participation in religious services.
5. Connectedness with a Higher Power is an important aspect of spirituality. While most choose to use God as their Higher Power, some people use other sources as their Higher Power.
6. Discuss recovery as a "we" rather than an "I" process. Emphasize the importance of looking beyond oneself and reaching out for help and support.
7. As recovery progresses, serving others is one way of expressing spirituality. Helping others is the basis of Step 12. However, this is only done after a substantial period of recovery.
8. Steps 2, 3, 5, 6, 7, 11, and 12 of the Twelve Step program address spirituality issues.
9. Ask clients to identify one area of spirituality they want to work on.
10. Discuss spirituality strategies to help recovery and personal growth. Strategies may include the following:
    - Rely on God or a Higher Power for strength, guidance, purpose in life, and understanding.
    - Participate in religious services and activities.
    - Make prayer a regular part of the day or join a prayer group.

- Attend a religious retreat or spend time at a monastery or other spiritual place to get in touch with spiritual beliefs.
- Meditate.
- Read the Bible or other spiritual and inspirational guides to seek knowledge, guidance, and motivation.
- Discuss spirituality issues in therapy sessions or with an AA/NA sponsor.
- Focus on Steps 2, 3, 5, 6, 7, 11, and 12.
- Seek spiritual advice from a priest, minister, rabbi, or other spiritual person.
- Focus on the greater good of society and contributions that can be made to make the world a better place.
- Be of service to others (volunteer work).
- Show love and compassion in daily life in interactions with other people.
- Be kind and forgiving to self and others.
- Accept one's weaknesses and limitations and be tolerant of shortcomings and mistakes.
- Stop hurtful behaviors toward others and make amends as needed.

Supporting Materials

Dennis C. Daley, *Dual Diagnosis Workbook: Recovery Strategies for Substance Use and Mental Health Disorders*, pp. 127–129. Independence, Missouri: Herald House/Independence Press, 2003.

Terence T. Gorski, *Keeping the Balance: A Psychospiritual Model of Growth and Development*. Independence, Missouri: Independence Press.

List of the Twelve Steps.

PE Group Topic #39
Using a Daily Plan in Recovery

Objectives

1. Review the importance of a daily plan in recovery.
2. Review ways to develop and use a daily plan.
3. Identify specific activities to include in a recovery plan.
4. Connect the idea of a daily recovery plan with the notion of a "daily inventory" stressed in Twelve Step programs of AA, NA, and DRA.

Points for Discussion

1. Ask clients why they think it is important to follow a daily plan in recovery. Add examples as needed to cover these benefits:
   - Helps keep clients focused and vigilant about recovery.
   - Keeps them busy and focused on using positive coping strategies.
   - Helps clients achieve their goals.
   - Helps them spot problems early.

2. Discuss the possible negative consequences of not following a recovery plan on a daily basis. Add examples as needed to cover the following potential problems:
   - Problems are not identified or addressed promptly.
   - Boredom and hopelessness are more likely.
   - Clients can lose focus on recovery.
   - Clients can become too passive about recovery and the actions needed to sustain recovery.
   - The risk of relapse may increase.

3. Ask clients what specific activities should be included in this daily plan. Emphasize the following (all won't be used every day):
   - Support group meetings (AA, NA, DRA, or mental health groups).
   - Discussion with sponsor or other members of support network.
   - Treatment sessions (individual, family, group).
   - Taking medication.
   - Working the Twelve Step program.

- Using other "tools" of the program (slogans, literature).
- Praying or using a Higher Power.
- Positive self-talk (to manage cravings, anger, anxiety, or depression).
- Challenging negative or inaccurate self-talk.
- Self-reflection (daily inventory, completion of daily journal entry).
- Reading recovery literature.
- Taking a few minutes at the beginning of each day to review and reflect on the day's recovery plan.
- Taking a few minutes at the end of the day to review and reflect on how things went and to identify early problems that need attention.

4. *Option:* discuss using a daily schedule and/or weekly schedule to help in this process. Provide samples of plans and blank planning schedules for clients to practice.

Supporting Materials

Dennis C. Daley, *Dual Diagnosis Workbook: Recovery Strategies for Substance Use and Mental Health Disorders*, pp. 132–134. Independence, Missouri: Herald House/Independence Press, 2003.

Blank copy of daily schedule.

Blank copy of weekly schedule.

PE Group Topic #40
Financial Issues in Dual Recovery

Objectives

1. Identify financial problems caused or worsened by substance use, psychiatric, or dual disorders.
2. Identify strategies to reduce debt.
3. Identify strategies to manage money more effectively.

Points for Discussion

1. Financial problems are associated with psychiatric, substance use, and dual disorders. Although any disorder can cause financial problems, substance use disorders and bipolar disorder often cause the most damage.
2. Financial problems can cause frustration, anger, and hopelessness for the client and family.
3. Ask clients to give examples of financial problems caused or worsened by their disorders. Include financial affects on the family and clients. Some of the more common problems include the following:
    - Using a paycheck, disability or government check, or other income to buy drugs or alcohol.
    - Loss of income due to inability to get or keep a job or being underemployed.
    - Inability to pay bills (rent, utilities) on time or meet basic needs for food, clothing, and shelter.
    - Inability to provide adequately for children or family (food, clothing, shelter, education).
    - Accumulating a large drug debt, which can put a client in danger due to retaliation by drug dealers.
    - Making bad investments, going on spending sprees, spending retirement income, or getting loans during periods of mania or hypomania.
    - Shopping excessively when depressed in an attempt to feel better.
    - Getting deeply into debt due to above problems or due to borrowing money at high rates of interest from financial institutions or loan sharks.
4. Review strategies to address client's financial problems and manage their money more effectively. Money-management strategies include the following:
    - Keeping track of money so clients know how they spend it.

- Developing and following a budget to live within financial means.
- Regularly reviewing progress and changing budget plan as needed.
- Reducing debts on loans and credit cards.
- Avoiding loan sharks and high interest loans.
- Shopping more effectively to stretch money.
- Figuring out "little ways" to save money here and there (adds up to substantial savings).
- Reading books and magazines to learn new ways of managing money.
- Seeking help from a financial counselor for money problems or financial consultant for investment advice.

5. Some clients may have no income at all. The goal with them is to find ways of financial support until they get back on their feet. This support may have to come initially from the government in the form of welfare. These clients may also benefit from information on food banks and other sources of help (help with utility payments).

Supporting Materials

Dennis C. Daley, *Dual Diagnosis Workbook: Recovery Strategies for Substance Use and Mental Health Disorders*, pp. 141–143. Independence, Missouri: Herald House/Independence Press, 2003.

Dennis C. Daley, *Money and Recovery Workbook*, 2nd ed. Holmes Beach, Florida: Learning Publications, 2001.

List of local resources and phone numbers (welfare office, food banks).

PE Group Topic #41
Managing Relapse Warning Signs

Objectives

1. Teach clients that warning signs precede a psychiatric or substance use relapse.
2. Introduce the idea that relapse is a process and an event.
3. Review common warning signs associated with psychiatric and substance use relapse.
4. Review subtle warning signs that may be unique to each individual.
5. Identify strategies to manage relapse warning signs.
6. For those who have had one or more episodes of relapse, teach them to use this as a learning experience to help their future recovery.

Points for Discussion

1. Ask clients to define relapse as it relates to the psychiatric and substance use disorders. Give the following definitions:
   - Psychiatric relapse refers to return of symptoms after a period of remission or a significant worsening of persistent symptoms.
   - Addiction relapse refers to the process of returning to alcohol or drug use after a period of sobriety.

2. Ask group members who have relapsed to either disorder for examples of relapse warning signs from past experiences. Add additional examples as needed and state that warning signs will fall in the following categories:
   - *Changes in thinking*: "I don't need recovery, it's not worth the effort, I don't need medications any more," increase in severity of paranoid thoughts, delusions, or hallucinations.
   - *Changes in mood*: significant increase in anger, anxiety, boredom, or depression.
   - *Changes in health habits or daily routines*: not taking care of personal hygiene or changes in daily habits or rituals.
   - *Changes in behavior*: stopping or cutting down on treatment sessions, medications, or support group meetings without prior discussion with a professional or AA, NA, or DRA sponsor; reducing social interactions or activities; or reduced use of the "tools of recovery."

3. For relapse to substance use, emphasize it seldom "comes out of the blue." Discuss the context of relapses (who, where, when) and help clients see that it may be days or longer between an emergence of warning signs and substance use.

4. Emphasize the importance of catching relapse warning signs early. The earlier that clients intervene, the less likely that relapse will occur.

5. Discuss the importance of not keeping warning signs a secret as things can build up and end in a relapse. Failure to identify or deal with relapse warning signs invites problems.

6. Ask clients to identify strategies to manage relapse warning signs. Their specific examples should fall in the following broad categories:

    - *Cognitive*: changing thoughts and beliefs (e.g., challenging the thought "I can't have fun without alcohol or drugs" or "Just because I didn't get the job I wanted doesn't mean I have to get depressed and give up").

    - *Behavioral*: changing a behavior (e.g., resuming regular meeting attendance when one identifies cutting back as a warning sign, taking medications as prescribed after one identifies cutting down or stopping without first discussing this with a doctor or therapist).

    - *Interpersonal*: seeking help and support from others in AA, NA, or DRA (e.g., talking with others about ways to manage warning signs).

7. Use this information to emphasize the importance of being aware of warning signs and having a plan to manage them.

8. Discuss the importance of seeking support from others to manage warning signs (e.g., AA/NA friends and sponsors, counselor, friends, family).

Supporting Materials

Dennis C. Daley, *Dual Diagnosis Workbook: Recovery Strategies for Substance Use and Mental Health Disorders*, pp. 149–153. Independence, Missouri: Herald House/Independence Press, 2003.

Dennis C. Daley, *Preventing Relapse Workbook*. Center City, Minnesota: Hazelden, 1993.

Dennis C. Daley, *Relapse Prevention Workbook*, 3rd ed. Holmes Beach, Florida: Learning Publications, 1999.

Terence T. Gorski, *Staying Sober*. Independence, Missouri: Independence Press, 1986.

Video: *Coping with Relapse Warning Signs,* 1994. Wilmette, Illinois: Gerald T. Rogers Productions. Phone: 1-800-227-9100; Web site: *www.gtrvideo.com*.

Video: *Developing a Relapse Plan*, 1995. Web site: *www.drdenniscdaley.com*.

Video: *Staying Sober, Keeping Straight*. Wilmette, Illinois: Gerald T. Rogers Productions. Phone: 1-800-227-9100; Web site: *www.gtrvideo.com*.

PE Group Topic #42
Managing High-Risk Relapse Factors

Objectives

1. Review factors that increase the risk of relapse to either disorder.
2. Label these as "high-risk" relapse factors.
3. Teach clients that relapse risk factors fall in different categories, and it is usually a combination of factors, rather than just one, that contribute to relapse.
4. Emphasize the importance of learning coping skills to manage relapse risk factors.
5. Identify strategies to manage high-risk relapse factors.

Points for Discussion

1. Relapse is common with psychiatric, substance use, and dual disorders. Relapse does not mean failure and is often part of a chronic or recurrent condition (medical, psychiatric, or addiction).
2. There are a number of external and internal factors that increase client's vulnerability to relapse. These are referred to as "high-risk" factors.
3. Ask group members to identify high-risk relapse factors in relation to their dual disorders.
4. Review the major categories of causes of relapse, giving some examples from each category:
   - Intrapersonal or internal factors (thoughts, feelings).
   - External factors (relationships, support system).
   - Lifestyle factors (health habits, structure).
5. Clients need more than awareness of their high-risk relapse factors. They also need coping skills to manage these effectively.
6. The skills needed vary and depend on the client's relapse risk factors.
7. Stress the importance of having a plan to deal with potential high-risk factors. The idea is to:
   - Identify (anticipate) high-risk factors.
   - Develop strategies to manage relapse-risk factors.
   - Implement coping strategies into daily recovery.
   - Change strategies that do not work and try new ones.

8. Reinforce the importance of making a commitment to long-term recovery using both professional counseling and self-help programs such as AA, NA, DRA, and mental health support groups. This provides an ongoing mechanism to identify and manage high-risk factors.

9. Some clients are more vulnerable to relapse than others, based on their history and severity of their illnesses and coping skills. For example:

    - A client with several episodes of depression is more vulnerable to a reoccurrence than a first-timer in treatment.

    - A client with a long history of addiction and multiple attempts at recovery is more vulnerable to relapse than a first timer.

Supporting Materials

Dennis C. Daley, *Preventing Relapse Workbook.* Center City, Minnesota: Hazelden, 1993.

Dennis C. Daley, *Relapse Prevention Workbook*, 3rd ed. Holmes Beach, Florida: Learning Publications, 1999.

Video: *Coping with Relapse Warning Signs,* 1994. Wilmette, Illinois: Gerald T. Rogers Productions. Phone: 1-800-227-9100; Web Site: *www.gtrvideo.com*.

Video: *Preventing Relapse.* Center City, Minnesota: Hazelden, 1994. Phone: 1-800-328-9000.

Video: *Staying Sober, Keeping Straight*. Wilmette, Illinois: Gerald T. Rogers Productions. Phone: 1-800-227-9100; Web Site: *www.gtrvideo.com*.

PE Group Topic #43
Coping with Emergencies and Setbacks

Objectives

1. Review the importance of being prepared to handle setbacks or emergencies (i.e., a return to substance use or a return or worsening of psychiatric symptoms).

2. Identify benefits of continued involvement in treatment and recovery.

3. Raise awareness that failure to comply with ongoing treatment increases the chance of relapse to either disorder.

Points for Discussion

1. Clients who comply with treatment do better than those who do not. Failure to comply with treatment often contributes to relapse.

2. Stress the importance of taking medications and keeping therapy appointments even after symptoms are under control or after sobriety has been achieved and maintained.

    - Medication and therapy can keep symptoms under control over the long term.

    - Medications reduce the likelihood of a psychiatric relapse or substance use relapse.

3. Ask clients who have failed to comply with treatment in the past, and those who did, to state how this affected their disorders and recovery.

4. Ask clients to identify the potential benefits of complying with treatment.

5. Many clients relapse, so it helps to be prepared should this occur. Relapse can occur even if clients comply with treatment. However it is less likely if treatment is complied with. Review the benefits of preparing ahead of time for a setback or relapse.

    - Clients are better prepared to take action quickly and early in the relapse process.

    - Clients feel more hopeful about recovery if they know how to handle setbacks and potential problems.

    - Damage that occurs following a relapse is limited.

6. Ask clients what they could do if they felt their treatment plan was not working or not helpful instead of dropping out of treatment.

    - Talk to their treatment team about changing the plan.

    - Talk to a sponsor.

    - Figure out why the plan is not working.

7. Ask clients to identify steps to take if they relapse to substance use.
   - Stop using and get rid of alcohol, drugs and drug paraphernalia.
   - Ask for help from a sponsor or other AA, NA, or DRA friends.
   - Ask for help from the treatment team.
   - Seek detoxification if physical addiction has reoccurred.
8. Review steps to take if psychiatric symptoms return or worsen. Emphasize the importance of talking with the treatment team and not keeping "secrets" regarding substance use, psychiatric symptoms, or poor adherence to treatment.
9. Encourage clients with a history of suicide attempts to develop a "safety contract" with their treatment team to help them intervene early should they feel suicidal.
10. Review the following ideas about setbacks and emergencies:
    - Preparing ahead of time allows clients to catch setbacks early, which may help prevent a full-blown relapse.
    - Clients can ask for help with setbacks or emergencies from counselors, other professionals, and sponsors.
    - When possible, the family should be involved.
    - Clients who decompensate psychiatrically and become suicidal, homicidal, or unable to care for themselves will probably need to be hospitalized. If they refuse, which is often due to poor judgment, an involuntary commitment may be needed.
    - Clients who get readdicted physically and cannot stop alcohol or drug use will need detoxified under medical supervision.

Supporting Materials

Dennis C. Daley, *Dual Diagnosis Workbook: Recovery Strategies for Substance Use and Mental Health Disorders*, pp. 154–156. Independence, Missouri: Herald House/Independence Press, 2003.

Dennis C. Daley, *Understanding Addiction and Suicide*. Center City, Minnesota: Hazelden, 2003.

Video: *Understanding Suicide and Addiction*, 2003. Center City, Minnesota: Hazelden. Web site: *www.hazelden.org*.

Endnotes

Chapter 1: Overview of Dual Disorders and Treatment

1. The Epidemiological Catchment Area study (Robins and Regier, 1991) and National Comorbidity study (Kessler et al., 1997) both document high rates of dual disorders. Many studies of clinical populations also document high rates of dual disorders. See notes 2 and 5 below for references that report prevalence data from clinical studies.

2. Many books have been published in the past decade that focus on integrated treatment for dual disorders. See CMHS, 1998; Daley and Moss, 2002; Daley and Zuckoff, 1999; Drake and Mueser, 1996; Minkoff and Drake, 1991; Montrose and Daley, 1995; Mercer-McFadden et al., 1998; Mueser et al., 1992, 1998, 1999, and 2002; O'Connell and Beyer, 2002; Onken et al., 1997b; Roberts and Shaner, 1999; Ryglewicz and Pepper, 1996; Salloum et al., 2000; USDHHS, 2002; and Westermeyer et al., 2003.

3. There are several comprehensive textbooks on addiction and many evidenced-based manuals and papers delineating specific treatments. See ASAM, 2003; APP, 1999; Beck et al., 1993; Daley, 2004; Daley and Marlatt, 1997b; Daley, Marlatt, and Spotts, 2003; Daley, Mercer, and Carpenter, 1998; Daley, Mercer, and Spotts, 2003; DeLeon, 2000; Higgins and Silverman, 1999; Lowinson et al., 1997; Marlatt and Gordon, 1985; McAullife and Albert, 1992; Meyers et al., 1999; Monti et al., 2002; NIAAA 1995a, b, c, and 1999; NIDA 1994, 1999a, b, c, d, 2000, 2002, and 2003; Obert et al., 2000; Project MATCH, 1998; Schuckit, 2002; The Matrix Center, 1989; Valasquez et al., 2002; and Washton, 1995.

4. There are several comprehensive textbooks on psychiatric disorders and many evidenced-based manuals and papers delineating specific treatments. Some approaches are adaptable to many types of disorders whereas others focus on one type of psychiatric illness. See Antony et al., 1997; Barlow et al., 1992; Beck, 1976; Beck et al., 2003; Bellack et al., 1997; Cloninger and Svrakic, 2000; Foa et al., 2000; Hogarty, 2002; Koerner and Linehan, 2000; Kozak and Foa, 1997; Kupfer et al., 1992; Liberman et al., 1989; Linehan, 1993; Miklowitz and Goldstein, 1997; Meuser and Glynn, 1999; Thase, 1999; Thase et al., 1994; Thase and Wright, 1991; Sadock and Sadock, 2000; Soloff, 1998 and 2000; and Weissman et al., 2000. See Kendall and Chambless, 1998, and Nathan and Gorman, 1998, for comprehensive reviews of empirical studies on specific treatments for various psychiatric disorders; see Hofmann and Tompson, 2002, for a review of empirically supported interventions for chronic and severe mental disorders; see Sammons and Schmidt, 2001, for a review of combined treatments; (psychological and pharmacological interventions) for psychiatric disorders; see APA, 1999, and Fink, 1999, for a review of electroconvulsive therapy (ECT).

5. In addition to the books listed in note 2 above, many chapters and journal articles focus on dual disorders. See Bellack and DiClemente, 1999; Bennet et al., 2001; Brady et al., 1994; Drake et al., 1993, 1996 and 1998; Gearon et al., 2001; Kaufman, 1989; Linehan et al., 1999; Longabaugh et al., 1995; Myrick and Brady, 1997;

Najavits and Weiss, 1998; Ridgely and Jerrell, 1996; Rosenthal and Westreich, 1999; Weiss et al., 2000.

6. Minkoff and Drake, 1991; and Drake and Mueser, 1996.
7. Mueser et al., 1998 and 2003; and Ridgely and Jerrell, 1996.
8. All of the major textbooks on addiction and psychiatric disorders discuss factors involved in the etiology of these disorders. For additional information on etiology, see Andreasen, 2001; Anthenelli and Schuckit, 1997; Cloninger, 1987; McLellan et al., 2000; O'Brien et al., 1998 Volkow and Fowler, 2000.
9. Meyer, 1986; Daley and Moss, 2002; Salloum and Thase, 2002.
10. Cloninger, 1987.
11. Daley, 1999; Daley and Zuckoff, 1999.
12. McLellan et al., 1983.
13. Catalano et al., 1988.
14. Bartels et al., 1995; Owen et al., 1997.
15. CMHS, 1998.
16. See references in notes 2, 3, 4, and 5 for evidenced-based treatments.
17. Daley and Zuckoff, 1998; Zweben and Zuckoff, 2003; Swanson et al., 2002.
18. Daley and Zuckoff, 1999.

Chapter 2: Recovery from Dual Disorders

1. See Daley, 2004, for a comprehensive review of recovery from dual disorders. See the AA "Big Book," NA "Basic Text," and the Dual Disorders Recovery Book for information on recovery using the Twelve Step model. Also, many workbooks published by Hazelden in the co-occurring disorders series provide a biopsychosocial framework for recovery from addiction combined with various types of psychiatric illness. For more detailed information about spirituality issues, see Enright and Fitzgibbons, 2000; McCullough, Pargament, and Thoresen, 2000; Richards and Bergin, 1997; Walsh, 1999; and White and MacDougall, 2001.
2. Prochaska et al., 1994.
3. Gorski, 1986; Marlatt and Gordon, 1985.
4. Thase, 1999.
5. Minkoff and Drake, 1991; Kaufman, 1989.

Chapter 3: Format of DDRC

1. Sammons and Schmidt, 2001.

2. Blackwell, 1997; Onken et al., 1997a; Petry and Bickel, 1999; Woody et al., 1985.

Chapter 5: The Assessment Process

1. APA, 2000a.
2. See Daley and Moss, 2002; Drake et al., 1998; and Mueser et al., 2003.
3. ASAM, 2001.
4. See Rosenberg et al., 1998 for a description of a questionnaire to assess substance use problems among clients with chronic mental disorders.
5. APA, 2000b.

Chapter 6: Motivation and Treatment Adherence

1. Miller and Rollnick, 2003; Daley and Zuckoff, 1999.
2. Bien et al., 1993.
3. Saunders et al., 1995.
4. Daley et al., 1998; Swanson et al., 2002; Zuckoff and Daley, 2001.
5. Mueser et al., 1992; Daley and Zuckoff, 1999.
6. Isenhart, 1994.
7. Longabaugh et al., 1995.
8. NIDA, 1991.
9. Hendriks, 1990.
10. Daley and Zuckoff, 1998.
11. Garbutt et al., 1999; Marmo and Holden, 1989; Daley and Marlatt, 1997a.
12. Greenstein et al., 1997.
13. Fram et al., 1989; Pristach and Smith, 1990.
14. Adams and Howe, 1993; Bebbington, 1995.
15. Swartz et al., 1998.
16. Carpenter et al., 1985; Casper and Donaldson, 1990; Havassy and Arns, 1998; Joyce, 1990; Keck et al., 1998; Kent and Yellowlees.
17. See Daley and Zuckoff, 1999, for a description of several applications of motivational strategies. See Miller and Rollnick, 2003, for a description of motivational interviewing and applications to multiple clinical populations. See also Bokos et al., 1992; Kadden and Mauriello, 1991; Simpson et al., 1997; Walitzer et al., 1999; Zweben and Zuckoff, 2003.

18. Drake et al., 1993; Moos et al., 1995; Peterson et al., 1994.
19. Owen et al., 1997; Walker et al., 1996; Verinis and Taylor, 1994.
20. Daley and Zuckoff, 1998; Wolpe et al., 1993.
21. Kemp et al., 1998.
22. Brown et al., 1995.
23. Hull et al., 1996; Joyce, 1990.
24. Olfson et al., 1998.
25. Daley and Zuckoff, 1998.
26. Swanson et al., 2002.
27. Haywood et al., 1995; Owen et al., 1997.
28. Joyce, 1990; Goodpastor and Hare, 1991; Geller, 1986.

Chapter 7: Individual Treatment

1. See note 4 in Chapter 1 on treatment of psychiatric disorders.
2. Sammons and Schmidt, 2001; Cornelius et al., 1997; Salloum et al., 1998 and 2000.
3. See note 3 in Chapter 1 on treatment of addictive disorders.
4. Payte et al., 2003; Stine et al., 2003.
5. Hurt et al., 2003; Daley and Marlatt, 1997b.
6. Saxon, 2003.
7. Pani et al., 2000; Payte et al., 2003; Stine et al., 2003.
8. Hurt et al., 2003.
9. Kranzler and Jaffe, 2003; NIAAA, 2000.
10. NIDA, 1999.
11. Daley and Zuckoff, 1999; Carey and Carey, 1990; Kadden and Mauriello, 1991; Ridgely and Willenbring, 1992.
12. Miller and Rollnick, 2002; NIAAA, 1995b.
13. Many of the references cited in Chapter 1 (see notes 2, 3, 4, and 5) report findings from empirical studies, which support the positive effects of various treatments.

Chapter 8: Role of the Family and Significant Others in Treatment

1. Daley and Miller, 2001; Daley and Spear, 2003; Hatfield and Lefley, 1987; Marsh and Dickens, 1997; Mueser and Ginerick, 1994; Torrey 2001 and 2002.

2. Effects of addiction on children are summarized in Daley and Miller, 2001. See also Moss et al., 1995a and b; Nunes et al., 2000; Tarter et al., 1995.

3. Daley and Moss, 2002.

4. Anderson et al., 1986; Glick et al., 2000; Hatfield, 1990; Johnson, 1989; McFarlane, 2002; Miklowitz and Goldstein, 1997; Mueser and Glynn, 1997; O'Farrell and Fals-Stewart, 1999; Stanton and Shadish, 1997.

Chapter 9: Overview of Group Treatments

1. Daley et al., 1998 and 2003b; Daley and Moss, 2002; The Matrix Center, 1989; Montrose and Daley, 1995; NIDA, 2002; Valasque et al., 2001; Washton, 1997; Yalom, 1985.

2. These are based on review of hundreds of videos of group treatment sessions in several clinical trials and observations of hundreds of treatment groups in many addiction and dual diagnosis treatment settings.

3. For a discussion of strategies to develop group programming, see Daley and Moss, 2003; Montrose and Daley, 1995.

Reference List

Adams, S.G., and J.T. Howe, Predicting medication compliance in a psychotic population. *The Journal of Nervous and Mental Disease*, 181 (9), 558–560, 1993.

Ahrens, C., J.W. Finney, R.H. Moos, P.C. and Ouimette, Posttraumatic stress disorder in substance abuse patients: Relationship to one-year posttreatment outcomes. *Psychology of Addictive Behaviors*, 11(1), 34–47, 1997.

America Psychiatric Association, The practice of electroconvulsive therapy: recommendations for treatment, training, and privileging. In: *A Task Force Report of the American Psychiatric Association*, Washington, D.C.: APA, 1999.

American Psychiatric Press, *Textbook of Substance Abuse Treatment*. McGalanter and H.D. Kleber, eds. Washington, D.C.: APP, 1999.

American Society on Addiction Medicine, *ASAM Patient Placement Criteria for the Treatment of Substance-Related Disorders*, 2nd ed. D. Mee-Lee, G.D. Shulman, M. Fishman, D.R. Gastfriend, J.H. Griffith, eds. Chevy Chase, Maryland: ASAM, 2001.

American Society on Addiction Medicine, *Principles of Addiction Medicine*, 3rd ed. A.W. Graham, T.K. Schultz, B.B. Wilford, eds. Chevy Chase, Maryland: ASAM, 2003.

Anderson, C.M., and S. Stewart, *Mastering Resistance*. New York: Guilford, 1984.

Anderson, C.M., D.J. Reiss, and G.E. Hogarty, *Schizophrenia and the Family*. New York: Guilford, 1986.

Andreasen, N.C., *Brave New Brain: Conquering Mental Illness in the Era of the Genome*. New York: Oxford University Press, 2001.

Anthenelli, R.M., and M.A. Schuckit, Genetics. In J.H. Lowinson, P. Ruiz, R.B. Millman, and J.G. Langrod, eds. *Substance Abuse: A Comprehensive Textbook*, 3rd ed. Baltimore, Maryland: Williams and Wilkins, 41–50, 1997.

Antony, M.M., D.H. Barlow, and M.G. Craske, *Mastery of Your Specific Phobia: Therapist Guide*. San Antonio, Texas: Psychological Corporation, 1997.

DSM-IV-TR: *Diagnostic and Statistical Manual of Mental Disorders* (revised edition). Washington, D.C.: APA, 2000a.

Handbook of Psychiatric Measures. Washington, D.C.: APA, 2000b.

Barlow, D.H., M.G. Craske, and T. O'Leary, *Mastery of Your Anxiety and Worry: Therapist Guide*. San Antonio, Texas: Psychological Corporation, 1992.

Bartels, S.J., R.E. Drake, and M.A. Wallach, Long-term course of substance use disorders among patients with severe mental illness. *Psychiatric Services*, 46 (3), 248–251, 1995.

Bebbington, P.E., The content and context of compliance. *International Clinical Psychopharmacology*, 9 (supp. 5), 41–50, 1995.

Beck, A.T., *Cognitive Therapy and the Emotional Disorders*. New York: New American Library, 1976.

Beck, A.T., A. Freeman, and Associates, *Cognitive Therapy of Personality Disorders*, 2nd ed. New York: Guilford, 2003.

Beck, A.T., F.D. Wright, C.F. Newman, and B.S. Liese, *Cognitive Therapy of Substance Abuse*. New York: Guilford, 1993.

Bellack, A.S., and C.C. DiClemente, Treating substance abuse among patients with schizophrenia. *Psychiatric Services* 50, 75–80, 1999.

Bellack, A.S., K.T. Mueser, S. Gingerich, and J. Agresta, *Social Skills Training for Schizophrenia: A Step-by-Step Guide*. New York: Guilford, 1997.

Bennet, M.E., A.S. Bellack, and J.S. Gearon, Treating substance abuse in schizophrenia. *Journal of Substance Abuse Treatment* 20, 163–175, 2001.

Bien, T.H., W.R. Miller, and J.S. Tonigan, Brief interventions for alcohol problems: A Review. *Addiction*, 88, 315–336, 1993.

Black, D.W., *Bad Boys, Bad Men: Confronting Antisocial Personality Disorder*. New York: Oxford University Press, 1999.

Blackwell, B., *Treatment Compliance and the Therapeutic Alliance*. The Netherlands: Harwood Academic Publishers, 1997.

Bokos, P.J., C.L. Metja, J.H. Michenberg, and R.L. Monks, Case management: an alternative approach to working with intravenous drug users. In R.S. Ashery, ed. *Progress and Issues in Case Management*. Rockville, Maryland: NIDA, 92–111, 1992.

Brady, K.T., T. Killeen, M.E. Saladin, B. Dansky, and S. Becker, Comorbid substance abuse and posttraumatic stress disorder: characteristics of women in treatment. *The American Journal on Addictions*, 3 (2), 160–164, 1994.

Brown, P.J., P.R. Recupero, and R. Stout, PTSD Substance abuse comorbidity and treatment utilization. *Addictive Behaviors*, 20 (2), 251–252, 1995.

Burns, D., *Ten Days to Self Esteem*. New York: Quill, 1993.

Carey, K.B., and M.P. Carey, Enhancing the treatment attendance of mentally ill chemical abusers. *Journal of Behavior Therapy and Experimental Psychiatry*, 21 (3), 205–209, 1990.

Carpenter, M.D., J.C. Mulligan, I.A. Bader, and A.E. Meinzer, Multiple admissions to an urban psychiatric center: a comparative study. *Hospital and Community Psychiatry*, 36 (12), 1305–1308, 1985.

Casper, E.S., and B. Donaldson, Subgroups in the population of frequent users of inpatient services. *Hospital and Community Psychiatry*, 41 (2), 189–191, 1990.

Catalano, R., M. Howard, J. Hawkins, and E. Wells, Relapse in the addictions: rates, determinants, and promising prevention strategies. In: *1988 Surgeon General's Report on Health Consequences of Smoking*. Washington, D.C.: Office of Smoking and Health, GPO, 1988.

Center for Mental Health Services. *Co-occurring Psychiatric and Substance Disorders in Managed Care Systems: Standards of Care, Practice Guidelines, Workforce Competencies, and Training Curricula*. Rockville, Maryland: CMHS, 1998.

Cloninger, C.R., Neurogenetic adaptive mechanisms in alcoholism. *Science*, 410–416, 1987.

Cloninger, C.R., and D.M. Svrakic, Personality disorders. In B.J. Sadock and V.A. Sadock, eds. *Comprehensive Textbook of Psychiatry*, 7th ed. Baltimore, Maryland: Lippincott, Williams, and Wilkins, 1723–1764, 2000.

Cornelius, J.R., I.M. Salloum, J.G. Ehler, et. al., Fluoxetine in depressed alcoholics. A double-blind, placebo-controlled trial. *Archives of General Psychiatry*, 54 (8), 700–705, 1997.

Craske, M.G., D.H. Barlow, and E. Meadows, *Mastery of Your Anxiety and Panic: Therapist Guide*, 3rd ed. San Antonio, Texas: Psychological Corporation, 2000.

Daley, D.C., A comparison of aftercare compliance and rehospitalization rates between psychiatric patients with and without comorbid substance use disorders. Pittsburgh, Pennsylvania: Author, 1999.

Daley, D.C., *Coping with Feelings Workbook*, 2nd ed. Holmes Beach, Florida: Learning Publications, 2003.

Daley, D.C., *Double Recovery: Managing Your Substance Use and Mental Health Disorders*. Memphis, Tennessee: Foundations, 2004.

Daley, D.C., *Dual Diagnosis Workbook: Recovery Strategies for Substance Use and Mental Health Problems*, 3rd ed. Independence, Missouri: Independence Press, 2003.

Daley, D.C., *Group Drug Counseling Manual for Bipolar Patients*. Pittsburgh, Pennsylvania: Author, 1999.

Daley, D.C., *Improving Communication and Relationships*. Holmes Beach, Florida: Learning Publications, 1996.

Daley, D.C., *Managing Anger Workbook*, 2nd ed. Holmes Beach, Florida: Learning Publications, 2001.

Daley, D.C., *Money and Recovery Workbook*, 2nd ed. Holmes Beach, Florida: Learning Publications, 2001.

Daley, D.C., *Overcoming Negative Thinking*. Center City, Minnesota: Hazelden, 1998.

Daley, D.C., *Preventing Relapse*, 2nd ed. Center City, Minnesota: Hazelden, 2003.

Daley, D.C., *Relapse Prevention: Treatment Models and Counseling Strategies*. Pittsburgh, Pennsylvania: Author, 2004.

Daley, D.C., *Relapse Prevention Workbook for Recovering Alcoholics and Drug Dependent Persons*, 3rd ed. Holmes Beach, Florida: Learning Publications, 2001.

Daley, D.C., *Understanding Addiction and Suicide*. Center City, Minnesota: Hazelden, 2003.

Daley, D.C., *Working through Denial*. Center City, Minnesota: Hazelden, 1998.

Daley, D.C., and R. Haskett, *Understanding Bipolar Disorder and Addiction*, 2nd ed. Center City, Minnesota: Hazelden, 2003.

Daley, D.C., and G.A. Marlatt, *Managing Your Drug or Alcohol Problem: Client Workbook*. San Antonio, Texas: Psychological Corporation, 1997a.

Daley, D.C., and G.A. Marlatt, *Managing Your Drug or Alcohol Problem: Therapist's Guide*. San Antonio, Texas: Psychological Corporation, 1997b.

Daley, D.C., G.A. Marlatt, and C. Spotts, Relapse prevention: clinical models and specific intervention strategies. In *Principles of Addiction Medicine*, 3rd ed. A.W. Graham, T.K. Schultz, and B.B. Wilford, eds. Chevy Chase, Maryland: American Society on Addiction Medicine, 467–486, 2003.

Daley, D.C., D. Mercer, and C. Spotts, Group treatment of substance use disorders. In A.W. Graham, F.K. Schultz, and B.B. Wilford, eds. *Principles of Addiction Medicine*, 3rd ed. Chevy Chase, Maryland: American Society on Addiction Medicine, 839–850, 2003.

Daley, D.C., D. Mercer, and G. Carpenter, *Group Drug Counseling Manual*. Holmes Beach, Florida: Learning Publications, 1998.

Daley, D.C., and J. Miller, *Addiction in Your Family: Helping Yourself and Your Loved Ones*. Holmes Beach, Florida: Learning Publications, 2001.

Daley, D.C., and K. Montrose, *Understanding Schizophrenia and Addiction*, 2nd ed. Center City, Minnesota: Hazelden, 2003.

Daley, D.C., and H.B. Moss, *Dual Disorders: Counseling Clients with Chemical Dependency and Mental Illness*, 3rd ed. Center City, Minnesota: Hazelden, 2002.

Daley, D.C., and I.M. Salloum, *Understanding Major Anxiety Disorders and Addiction*, 2nd ed. Center City, Minnesota: Hazelden, 2003.

Daley, D.C., I.M. Salloum, A. Zuckoff, L. Kirisci, and M.E. Thase, Increasing treatment compliance among outpatients with depression and cocaine dependence. Results of a pilot study. *American Journal of Psychiatry*, 155, 1611–1613, 1998.

Daley, D.C., and J. Sinberg-Spear, *A Family Guide to Coping with Dual Disorders*, 3rd ed. Center City, Minnesota: Hazelden, 2003.

Daley, D.C., and M.E. Thase, *Understanding Depression and Addiction*, 2nd ed. Center City, Minnesota: Hazelden, 2003.

Daley, D.C., and A. Zuckoff, Improving compliance with the initial outpatient session among discharged inpatient dual diagnosis clients. *Social Work*, 43, 385–480, 1998.

Daley, D.C., and A. Zuckoff, *Improving Treatment Compliance: Counseling and System Strategies for Substance Use and Dual Disorders*. Center City, Minnesota: Hazelden, 1999.

DeLeon, G., *The Therapeutic Community: Theory, Model and Method*. New York: Springer Publications, 2000.

Drake, R.E., G.J. McHugo, and D.J. Noordsy, Treatment for alcoholism among schizophrenic outpatients: four-year outcomes. *American Journal of Psychiatry*, 150 (2), 328–329, 1993.

Drake, R.E., C. Mercer-McFadden, K.T. Mueser, G. McHugho, and G. Bond, A review of integrated mental health and substance abuse treatment for patients with dual disorders. *Schizophrenia Bulletin*, 24, 589–608, 1998.

Drake, R.E., K.T. Mueser, R.E. Clark, and M.A. Wallach, The course, treatment, and outcome of substance disorder in persons with severe mental illness. *American Journal of Orthopsychiatry*, 66 (1), 42–51, 1996.

Drake, R.E., and K.T. Mueser, eds., *Dual Diagnosis of Major Mental Illness and Substance Abuse*. San Francisco: Jossey-Bass, 1996.

Drake, R.E., and K.T. Mueser, Psychosocial approaches to dual diagnosis. *Schizophrenia Bulletin*, 26 (1), 105–118, 2000.

The Dual Disorders Recovery Book, Center City, Minnesota: Hazelden, 1993.

Edwards, M.R., and P. Steinglass, Family therapy treatment outcomes for alcoholism. *Journal of Marital and Family Therapy*, 21 (4), 475–509, 1995.

Enright, R.B., and R.P. Fitzgibbons, *Helping Clients Forgive: An Empirical Guide for Resolving Anger and Restoring Hope*. Washington, D.C.: APA, 2000.

Fink, M., *Electroshock: Restoring the Mind*. New York: Oxford University Press, 1999.

Fisher, M.S., and K.J. Bentley, Two group therapy models for clients with a dual diagnosis of substance abuse and personality disorder. *Psychiatric Services*, 47 (11), 1244–1250, 1996.

Foa, E.B., T.M. Keane, and M.J. Friedman, eds., *Effective Treatments of PTSD*. New York: Guilford, 2000.

Fram, D.H., J. Marmo, and R. Holden, Naltrexone treatment: the problem of patient acceptance. *Journal of Substance Abuse Treatment*, 6, 119–122, 1989.

Garbutt, J.C., S.L. West, T.S. Carey, K.N. Lohr, and F.T. Crews, Pharmacological treatment of alcohol dependence: A review of the evidence. *Journal of the American Medical Association*, 281 (14), 1318–1325, 1999.

Garrett, J., J. Landau-Stanton, M.D. Stanton, J. Stellato-Kabat, and D. Stellato-Kabat, ARISE: A method for engaging reluctant alcohol- and drug-dependent individuals in treatment. *Journal of Substance Abuse Treatment*, 14 (3), 235–248, 1997.

Gearon, J.S., A.S. Bellack, J. Rachbeisel, and L. Dixon, Drug-use behavior and correlates in people with schizophrenia. *Addictive Behaviors*, 26, 51–61, 2001.

Geller, J.L., In again, out again: Preliminary evaluation of a state hospital's worst recidivists. *Hospital and Community Psychiatry*, 37, 386–390, 1986.

Giancola, P., C. Martin, R. Tarter, H. Moss, and W. Pelham, Executive cognitive functioning and aggressive behavior in preadolescent boys at high risk for substance abuse. *Journal of Studies on Alcohol*, 57, 352–359, 1996.

Glick, I.D., E.M. Berman, J.F. Clarkin, and D.S. Rait, *Marital and Family Therapy*, 4th ed. Washington, D.C.: APA, 2000.

Goldstein, M.J., Psychosocial strategies for maximizing the effects of psychotropic medications for schizophrenia and mood disorder. *Psychopharmacology Bulletin*, 28, 237–240, 1992.

Goodpastor, W.A., and H.K. Hare, Factors associated with multiple readmissions to an urban public psychiatric hospital. *Hospital and Community Psychiatry*, 42 (1), 85–87, 1991.

Gorski, T.T., *Denial Management Counseling: Professional Guide*. Independence, Missouri: Independence Press, 2000.

Gorski, T.T., *Denial Management Counseling Workbook*. Independence, Missouri: Independence Press, 2000.

Gorski, T.T., *Getting Love Right*. New York, New York: Fireside/Parkside, 1993.

Gorski, T.T., *Staying Sober*. Independence, Missouri: Independence Press, 1986.

Greenstein, R.A., P.J. Fudala, and C.P. O'Brien, Alternative pharmacotherapies for opiate addiction. In J. H. Lowinson, P. Ruiz, R. B. Millman, and J. G. Langrod, eds., *Substance Abuse: A Comprehensive Textbook*, 3rd ed. Baltimore, Maryland: Lippincott, Williams and Wilkins, 415–424, 1997.

Hatfield, A.B., *Family Education in Mental Illness*. New York: Guilford, 1990.

Hatfield, A.B., and H.P. Lefley (eds.), *Families of the Mentally Ill: Coping and Adaptation*. New York: Guilford, 1987.

Havassy, B.E., and P.G. Arns, Relationship of cocaine and other substance dependence to well-being of high-risk psychiatric patients. *Psychiatric Services*, 49, 935–940, 1998.

Haywood, T.W., H.M. Kravitz, L.S. Grossman, J.L. Cavanaugh, J.M. Davis, and D.A. Lewis, Predicting the "revolving door" phenomenon among patients with schizophrenic, schizoaffective, and affective disorders. *American Journal of Psychiatry*, 152 (6), 856–861, 1995.

Hendin, H., and J.J. Mann, eds., The clinical science of suicide prevention. *Annals of the New York Academy of Sciences*, 932, 1–240, 2001.

Hendriks, V.M., *Addiction and Psychopathology: A Multidimensional Approach to Clinical Practice*. Rotterdam, The Netherlands: European Addiction Research Institute, 1990.

Higgins, S.T., and K. Silverman, eds., Motivating Behavior Change among Illicit Drug Abusers: Research on Contingency Management. Washington, D.C.: APA, 1999.

Hill, S.Y., M.D. DeBellis, M.S. Keshavan, L. Lowers, S. Shen, J. Hall, and T. Pitts, Right amygdala volume in adolescent and young adult offspring from families at high risk for developing alcoholism. *Society of Biological Psychiatry*, 49, 894–905, 2001.

Hogarty, G.E., *Personal Therapy: A Guide to the Individual Treatment of Schizophrenia and Related Disorders*. New York: Guilford, 2002.

Hull, J.W., F. Yeomans, J. Clarkin, C. Li, and G. Goodman, Factors associated with multiple hospitalization of patients with borderline personality disorder. *Psychiatric Services*, 47, 638–641, 1996.

Hurt, R.D., J.O. Ebbert, J.T. Hays, and L.C. Dale, Pharmacologic interventions for tobacco dependence. In *American Society on Addiction Medicine* (ASAM). *Principles of Addiction Medicine*, 3rd ed. A.W. Graham, T.K. Schultz, B.B. Wilford (eds.). Chevy Chase, Maryland: ASAM, 801–814, 2003.

Isenberg, K.E., and C.F. Zorumski, Electroconvulsive therapy. In B. J. Sadock, and V. A. Sadock, eds., *Comprehensive Textbook of Psychiatry*, 7th ed. New York: Lippincott Williams and Wilkins, 2503–2515, 2000.

Isenhart, C.F., Motivational subtypes in an inpatient sample of substance abusers. *Addictive Behaviors*, 19 (5), 463–475, 1994.

Jacob, R.G., and W.H. Pelham, Behavior therapy. In: B.J. Sadock and V.A. Sadock, eds., *Comprehensive Textbook of Psychiatry*, 7th ed. Baltimore, Maryland: Lippincott Williams and Wilkins, 2080–2127, 2000.

Johnson, V., *Intervention: How to Help Someone Who Doesn't Want Help*. Minneapolis, Minnesota: Johnson Institute, 1989.

Joyce, L.T., The new revolving-door patients: Results from a national cohort of first admissions. *Acta Psychiatric Scandinavia*, 82, 130–135, 1990.

Kadden, R.M., and I.J. Mauriello, Enhancing participation in substance abuse treatment using an incentive system. *Journal of Substance Abuse Treatment*, 8, 113–124, 1991.

Kaufman, E., The psychotherapy of dually diagnosed clients. *Journal of Substance Abuse Treatment*, 6, 9–18, 1989.

Keck, P.E., S.L. McElroy, S.M. Strakowski, S.A. West, K.W. Sax, J.M. Hawkins, M.L. Bourne, and P. Haggard, Twelve-month outcome of patients with bipolar disorder following hospitalization for a manic or mixed episode. *American Journal of Psychiatry*, 55 (5), 646–652, 1998.

Kemp, A., G. Kirov, B. Everitt, P. Kayward, and A. David, Randomized controlled trial of compliance therapy. *British Journal of Psychiatry*, 172, 413–419, 1998.

Kendall, P.C., and D.L. Chambless, eds., Empirically supported psychological therapies. *Journal of Consulting and Clinical Psychology*, 66, 1–209, 1998.

Kent, S., and P. Yellowlees, Psychiatric and social reasons for frequent rehospitalization. *Hospital and Community Psychiatry*, 45, 347–350, 1994.

Kessler, R.C., R.M. Crum, L.A. Warner, C.B. Nelson, J. Schulenberg, and J.C. Anthony, Lifetime co-occurrence of DSM-III-R alcohol abuse and dependence with other psychiatric disorders in the National Comorbidity Survey. *Archives of General Psychiatry*, 54, 313–321, 1997.

Koerner, K., and M.M. Linehan, Research on dialectical behavior therapy for patients with borderline personality disorder. *The Psychiatric Clinics of North America*, 23 (1), 151–167, 2000.

Kozak, M.J., and E.B. Foa, *Mastery of Obsessive–Compulsive Disorder: A Cognitive-Behavioral Approach: Therapist Guide*. San Antonio, Texas: Psychological Corporation, 1997.

Kranzler, H.R., and J.H. Jaffe, Pharmacologic interventions for alcoholism. In American Society on Addiction Medicine (ASAM). *Principles of Addiction Medicine*, 3rd ed. A.W. Graham, T.K. Schultz, B.B. Wilford, eds. Chevy Chase, Maryland: ASAM, 701–720, 2003.

Kupfer, D.J., E. Frank, J.M. Perel, et al., Five-year outcome for maintenance therapies in recurrent depression. *Archives of General Psychiatry*, 49, 769–773, 1992.

LaBounty, L.P., D. Hatsukami, S.F. Morgan, and L. Nelson, Relapse among alcoholics with phobic and panic symptoms. *Addictive Behaviors*, 17 (1), 9–15, 1992.

Liberman, R.P., *Social and Independent Living Skills Symptom Management Module*. Los Angeles, California: UCLA Department of Psychiatry, 1988.

Liberman, R.P., W.J. DeRisi, and K.T. Mueser, *Social Skills Training for Psychiatric Patients*. New York: Pergamon Press, 1989.

Linehan, M.M., *Cognitive–Behavioral Treatment of Borderline Personality Disorder*. New York: Guilford, 1993.

Linehan, M.M., H. Scmidt III, L.A. Dimeff, J.C. Craft, J. Kanter, and K.A. Comtois, Dialectical behavior therapy for patients with borderline personality disorder and drug-dependence. *The American Journal on Addictions*, 8, 279–292, 1999.

Longabaugh, R., A. Rubin, P. Malloy, M. Beattie, P.R. Clifford, and N. Noel, Drinking outcomes of alcohol abusers diagnosed as antisocial personality disorder. *Alcoholism: Clinical and Experimental Research*, 18 (4), 778–785, 1995.

Lowinson, J.H., P. Ruiz, R.B. Millman, and J.G. Langrod, eds., *Substance Abuse: A Comprehensive Textbook*, 3rd ed. Baltimore, Maryland: Williams and Wilkins, 1997.

Marlatt, G.A., and J.R. Gordon, eds., *Relapse Prevention: Maintenance Strategies in the Treatment of Addictive Behaviors*. New York: Guilford, 1985.

Marmo, J., and R. Holden, Naltrexone treatment—the problem of patient acceptance. *Journal of Substance Abuse Treatment*, 5, 199–122, 1989.

Marsh, D., and R. Dickens, *How to Cope with Mental Illness in Your Family*. New York: J.P. Tarcher, 1998.

Martin, C., M. Earleywine, T. Blackson, M. Vanyukov, H. Moss, and R. Tarter, Aggressivity, inattention, hyperactivity, and impulsivity in boys at high and low risk for substance abuse. *Journal of Abnormal Child Psychology*, 22, 177–203, 1994.

The Matrix Center, *The Neurobehavioral Treatment Model*, volumes I and II. Beverly Hills, California: The Matrix Center, 1989.

McAuliffe, W.E., and J. Albert, *Clean Start: An Outpatient Program for Initiating Cocaine Recovery*. New York: Guilford, 1992.

McCrady, B.S., Extending relapse prevention to couples. *Addictive Behaviors*, 14, 69–74, 1989.

McCullough, M.E., K.I. Pargament, and C.E. Thoresen, eds., *Forgiveness: Theory, Research and Practice*. New York: Guilford, 2000.

McFarlane, W.R., *Multifamily Groups in the Treatment of Severe Psychiatric Disorders*. New York: Guilford, 2002.

McKay, J.R., Studies of factors of relapse to alcohol, drug, and nicotine use: a critical review of methodologies and findings. *Journal of Studies on Alcohol*, 60, 566–576, 1999.

McLellan, A.T., *Guide to the Addiction Severity Index*. Rockville, Maryland: NIDA, 1985.

McLellan, A.T., D.C. Lewis, C.P. O'Brien, and H.D. Kleber, Drug dependence, a chronic medical illness: Implications for treatment, insurance, and outcomes evaluation. *Journal of the American Medical Association*, 284 (13), 1689–1695, 2000.

McLellan, A.T., L. Luborsky, and G.E. Woody, Predicting response to alcohol and drug abuse treatment. *Archives of General Psychiatry*, 40, 620–625, 1983.

Mercer-McFadden, C., R.E. Drake, R.E., Clark, et al., *Substance Abuse Treatment for People with Severe Mental Disorders: A Program Manager's Guide*. Dartmouth, New Hampshire: New Hampshire–Dartmouth Psychiatric Research Center, 1998.

Meyer, R., ed., *Addictive Disorders and Psychopathology*. New York: Guilford, 1986.

Meyers, R.J., W.R. Miller, D.E. Hill, and J.S. Tonigan, Community reinforcement and family training. *Journal of Substance Abuse Treatment*, 10 (3), 291–308, 1999.

Miklowitz, D.K., and M.J. Goldstein, *Bipolar Disorder: A Family-focused Treatment Approach*. New York: Guilford, 1997.

Miller, W.R., *Integrating Spirituality into Treatment: Resources for Practitioners*. Washington, D.C.: APA, 1999.

Miller, W.R., and S. Rollnick, *Motivational Interviewing: Preparing People to Change Addictive Behavior*, 2nd ed. New York: Guilford, 2003.

Millon, T., *Disorders of Personality*. New York: John Wiley and Sons, 1980.

Miner, C.R., R.N. Rosenthal, D.J. Hellerstein, and L.R. Muenz, Prediction of compliance with outpatient referral in patients with schizophrenia and psychoactive substance use disorders. *Archives of General Psychiatry*, 54, 706–712, 1997.

Minkoff, K., and R.E. Drake, eds., *Dual Diagnosis of Major Mental Illness and Substance Disorders*. San Francisco: Jossey-Bass, 1991.

Monti, P., D. Adams, R. Kadden, N. Cooney, and D. Abrams, *Treating Alcohol Dependence*. New York: Guilford, 2002

Montimore, F.M., *Bipolar Disorder: A Guide for Patients and Families*. Baltimore, Maryland: Johns Hopkins Press, 1999.

Montrose, K., and D.C. Daley, *Celebrating Small Victories: Treating Chronic Mental Illness and Substance Abuse*. Center City, Minnesota: Hazelden, 1995.

Moos, R.H., B. Pettit, and V. Gruber, Longer episodes of community residential care reduce substance abuse patients' readmission rates. *Journal of Studies on Alcohol*, 56, 433–443, 1995.

Moss, H., A. Mezzich, J. Yao, J. Gavaler, and C. Martin, Aggressivity among sons of substance abusing fathers: Association with psychiatric disorder in the father and son, paternal personality, pubertal development, and socioeconomic status. *The American Journal of Drug and Alcohol Abuse*, 21, 195–208, 1995a.

Moss, H., M. Vanyukov, P. Majumder, L. Kirisci, and R. Tarter, Perpubertal sons of substance abusers: Influences of parental and familial substance abuse on behavioral disposition, IQ, and school achievement. *Addictive Behaviors*, 20, 1–14, 1995b.

Mueser, K.T., A.S. Bellack, and J.J. Blanchard, Comorbidity of schizophrenia and substance abuse: Implications for treatment. *Journal of Consulting and Clinical Psychology*, 60 (6), 845–856, 1992.

Mueser, K.T., R.E. Drake, R. Clark, R., et al., *Toolkit: Evaluating Substance Abuse in Persons with Severe Mental Illness*. Dartmouth, New Hampshire: New Hampshire–Dartmouth Psychiatric Research Center, 1995.

Mueser, K.T., R.E. Drake, and D.L. Noordsy, Integrated mental health and substance abuse treatment for severe psychiatric disorders. *Journal of Practical Psychiatry and Behavioral Health*, 4 (3), 129–139, 1998.

Mueser, K.T., and K. Ginerick, *Coping with Schizophrenia: A Guide for Families*. Oakland, California: New Harbinger, 1994.

Mueser, K.T., and S.M. Glynn, *Behavioral Family Therapy for Psychiatric Disorders*, 2nd ed. Oakland, California: New Harbinger, 1999.

Mueser, K.T., D.L. Noordsy, R.E. Drake, and L. Fox, *Integrated Treatment for Dual Disorders: A Guide to Effective Practice*. New York: Guilford, 2003.

Myrick, H., and K.T. Brady, Social phobia in cocaine-dependent individuals. *The American Journal on Addictions*, 6 (2), 99–104, 1997.

Najavits, L.M., and R.D. Weiss, "Seeking safety" outcome of a new cognitive-behavioral psychotherapy for women with posttraumatic stress disorder and substance dependence. *Journal of Traumatic Stress*, 11, 437–456, 1998.

Nathan, P.E., and J.M. Gorman, eds., *A Guide to Treatments That Work*, 2nd ed. New York: Oxford University Press, 2002.

NIAAA, *Alcohol and Health: Tenth Special Report to the U.S. Congress*. Rockville, Maryland: USDHHS, 2000.

NIAAA, Project Match Series, volume 1. *Twelve Step Facilitation Therapy Manual*. Rockville, Maryland: USDHHS, 1995a.

NIAAA, Project Match Series, volume 2. *Motivational Enhancement Therapy Manual*. Rockville, Maryland: USDHHS, 1995b.

NIAAA, Project Match Series, volume 3. *Cognitive-Behavioral Coping Skills Therapy Manual*. Rockville, Maryland: USDHHS, 1995c.

NIAAA, Update on approaches to alcoholism treatment. *Alcohol Research and Health*, 23 (2), 1999.

NIDA, *Addict Aftercare: Recovery Training and Self-Help*, 2nd ed. Rockville, Maryland: NIDA, 1994.

NIDA, *Approaches to Drug Abuse Treatment*. Rockville, Maryland: NIDA, 2000.

NIDA, Drug abuse and psychiatric illness. *In Drug Abuse and Drug Abuse Research*. Rockville, Maryland: NIDA, 61–83, 1991.

NIDA, *Principles of Drug Addiction Treatment: A Research-Based Guide*. Rockville, Maryland: NIDA, 1999.

NIDA, Study sheds new light on the state of drug abuse treatment nationwide. *NIDA Notes*, 12 (5), 1–8, 1997.

NIDA, *Therapy Manuals for Drug Addiction, Manual 1. A Cognitive Behavioral Approach: Treating Cocaine Addiction*. Rockville, Maryland: USDHHS, 1998.

NIDA, *Therapy Manuals for Drug Addiction, Manual 2. A Community Reinforcement Plus Vouchers Approach: Treating Cocaine Addiction*. Rockville, Maryland: USDHHS, 1998.

NIDA, *Therapy Manuals for Drug Addiction, Manual 3*. An individual drug counseling approach to treat cocaine addiction. Rockville, Maryland: USDHHS, 1999.

NIDA, *Therapy Manuals for Drug Addiction, Manual 4. A Group Drug Counseling Approach to Treat Cocaine Addiction*. Rockville, Maryland: USDHHS, 2002.

NIDA, *Therapy Manuals for Drug Addiction, Manual 5. Multi-Systemic Family Therapy*. Rockville, Maryland: USDHHS, 2004.

Nunes, E.V., M.M. Weissman, R. Goldstein, et al., Psychiatric disorders and impairment in the children of opiate addicts: Prevalences and distribution by ethnicity. *American Journal on Addictions*, 9, 232–241, 2000.

Obert, J.L., M.J. McCann, P. Marinelli-Casey, A. Weiner, S. Minsky, P. Brethen, P., and R. Rawson, The matrix model of outpatient stimulant abuse treatment: History and description. *Journal of Psychoactive Drugs*, 32 (2), 157–164, 2000.

O'Brien, C.P., A.R. Childress, R. Ehrman, and S.J. Robbins, Conditioning factors in drug abuse: Can they explain compulsion? *Psychopharmacology*, 12, 15–22, 1998.

O'Connell, D., and E. Beyer, eds., *Managing the Dually Diagnosed Patient*, 2nd ed. New York: Haworth, 2002.

O'Farrell, T.J., and W. Fals-Stewart, Treatment models and methods: Family models. In B.S. McCrady and E.E. Epstein, eds., *Addictions: A Comprehensive Guidebook*. London: Oxford University Press, 287–305, 1999.

Olfson, M., D. Mechanic, C.A. Boyer, and S. Hansell, Linking inpatients with schizophrenia to outpatient care. *Psychiatric Services*, 49 (7), 911–917, 1998.

Onken, L.S., J.D. Blaine, and J. Boren, eds., *Beyond the Therapeutic Alliance: Keeping the Drug-dependent Individual in Treatment*. NIDA Research Monograph 165. Rockville, Maryland: USDHHS, 1997a.

Onken, L.S., J.D. Blaine, S. Genser, and A.M. Horton, *Treatment of Drug-Dependent Individuals with Comorbid Mental Disorders*. Rockville, Maryland: USDHHS, 1997b.

Osher, F.C., and L.L. Kofoed, Treatment of patients with psychiatric and psychoactive substance use disorders. *Hospital and Community Psychiatry*, 40, 1025–1030, 1989.

Owen, C., V. Rutherford, M. Jones, C. Tennant, and M.B. Smallman, International update: Psychiatric rehospitalization following hospital discharge. *Community Mental Health Journal*, 33, 13–22, 1997.

Owen, C., V. Rutherford, M. Jones, C. Tennant, and A. Smallman, Noncompliance in psychiatric aftercare. *Community of Mental Health Journal*, 33 (1) 25–34, 1997.

Pani, P.P., I. Maremmani, R. Pirastu, A. Tagliamonte, and G. Luigi-Gessa, Buprenorphine: a controlled clinical trial in the treatment of opioid dependence. *Drug and Alcohol Dependence*, 60, 39–50, 2000.

Payte, J.T., J.E. Zweben, and J. Martin, Opioid maintenance treatment. In *American Society on Addiction Medicine* (ASAM). *Principles of Addiction Medicine*, 3rd ed. A.W. Graham, T.K. Schultz, B.B. Wilford, eds. Chevy Chase, Maryland: ASAM, 751–766, 2003.

Peterson, K.A., R.W. Swindle, C.S. Phibbs, B. Recine, and R.H. Moos, Determinants of readmission following inpatient substance abuse treatment: A national study of VA programs. *Medical Care*, 32, 535–550, 1994.

Petry, N.M., and W.K. Bickel, Therapeutic alliance and psychiatric severity as predictors of completion of treatment for opioid dependence. *Psychiatric Services*, 50 (2), 219–227, 1999.

Pristach, A., and C.M. Smith, Medication compliance and substance abuse among schizophrenic patients. *Hospital and Community Psychiatry*, 41 (12), 1345–1348, 1990.

Prochaska, J.O., J.C. Norcross, and C.C. DiClemente, *Changing for Good*. New York: William Morrow, 1994.

Project MATCH, Matching alcoholism treatments to client heterogeneity: Project MATCH three-year drinking outcomes. *Alcoholism: Clinical and Experimental Research*, 22 (6), 1300–1311, 1998.

Richards, P.S., and A.E. Bergin, *A Spiritual Strategy for Counseling and Psychotherapy*. Washington, D.C.: APA, 1997.

Ridgely, M.S., and J.M. Jerrell, Analysis of three interventions for substance abuse treatment of severely mentally ill people. *Community Mental Health Journal*, 32 (6), 561–572, 1996.

Ridgely, M.S., and W.L. Willenbring, Application of case management to drug abuse treatment: Overview of models and research issues. In: *Progress and Issues in Case Management*. R.S. Ashery, ed. Rockville, Maryland: NIDA, 12–33, 1992.

Roberts, L.J., A. Shaner, and T.A. Eckman, *Overcoming Addictions: Skills Training for People with Schizophrenia*. New York: Norton, 1999.

Robins, L.N., and D.A. Regier, *Psychiatric Disorders in America*. New York: Free Press, 1991.

Rosenberg, S.D., R.E. Drake, G.L. Wolford, K.T. Meuser, T.E. Oxman, R.M. Vidaver, K.L. Carrieri, and R. Luckoor, The Dartmouth assessment of lifestyle instrument (DALI): A substance abuse disorder screen for people with severe mental illness. *American Journal of Psychiatry*, 155, 232–238, 1998.

Rosenthal, R.N., and L. Westreich, Treatment of persons with dual diagnosis of substance use disorder and other psychological problems. In B.S. McCrady and E.E. Epstein, eds., *Addictions: A Comprehensive Guidebook*. New York: Oxford University Press, 439–76, 1999.

Ryglewicz, H., and B. Pepper, *Lives at Risk: Understanding and Treating Young People with Dual Disorders*. New York: Free Press, 1996.

Sadock, B.J., and V.A. Sadock, eds., *Comprehensive Textbook of Psychiatry*, 7th ed. Baltimore, Maryland: Lippincott, Williams and Wilkins, 2000.

Salloum, I.M., J.R. Cornelius, M.E. Thase, D.C. Daley, L. Kirisci, and C.E. Spotts, Naltrexone utility in depressed alcoholics. *Psychopharmacology Bulletin*, 34 (1), 111–115, 1998.

Salloum, I.M., D.C. Daley, and M.E. Thase, *Male Depression, Alcoholism, and Violence*. London, United Kingdom: Martin Dunitz, 2000.

Salloum, I.M., and M.E. Thase, Impact of substance abuse on the course and treatment of bipolar disorder. *Bipolar Disorders*, 2, 2269–2280, 2000.

Saunders, B., C. Wilkinson, and M. Phillips, The impact of a brief motivational intervention with opiate users attending a methadone programme. *Addiction*, 90, 415–424, 1995.

Saxon, A.J., Special issues in office based opioid treatment. In *American Society on Addiction Medicine* (ASAM). *Principles of Addiction Medicine*, 3rd ed. A.W. Graham, T.K. Schultz, B.B. Wilford, eds. Chevy Chase, Maryland: ASAM, 767–784, 2003.

Shea, S.C., *The Practical Art of Suicide Assessment: A Guide for Mental Health Professionals and Substance Abuse Counselors*. New York: John Wiley, 1999.

Simpson, D.D., G.W. Joe, G.A. Rowan-Szal, and J.M. Greener, Drug abuse treatment process components that improve retention. *Journal of Substance Abuse Treatment*, 14 (6), 565–572, 1997.

Soloff, P., Algorithms for pharmacological treatment of personality dimensions: Symptom-specific treatments for cognitive-perceptual, affective, and impulsive-behavioral dysregulation. *Bulletin of the Menninger Clinic*, 62 (2), 195–214, 1998.

Soloff, P., Psychopharmacology of borderline personality disorder. *The Psychiatric Clinics of North America*, 23 (1), 169–192, 2000.

Stanton, M.D., and W.R. Shadish, Outcome, attrition, and family-couples treatments for drug abuse: A meta-analysis and review of the controlled, comparative studies. *Psychological Bulletin*, 122 (2), 170–191, 1997.

Stine, S.M., M.K. Greenwald, and T.R. Kosten, Pharmacologic interventions for opioid addiction. In *American Society on Addiction Medicine* (ASAM). *Principles of Addiction Medicine*, 3rd ed. A.W. Graham, T.K. Schultz, B.B. Wilford, eds. Chevy Chase, Maryland: ASAM, 735–748, 2003.

Sullivan, J.T., K. Sykora, J. Schneiderman, C.A. Naranjo, and E.M. Sellers, Assessment of alcohol withdrawal: the revised clinical institute withdrawal assessment for alcohol scale (CIWA-Ar). *British Journal of Addiction*, 84, 1353–1357, 1989.

Swanson, A.J., M.V. Pantalon, and R.K. Cohen, Motivational interviewing and treatment adherence among psychiatric and dually diagnosed patients. *Journal of Nervous and Mental Disease*, 187, 630–635, 2002.

Swartz, M.S., J.W. Swanson, V.A. Hiday, R. Borum, H.R. Wagner, and B.J. Burns, Violence and severe mental illness: The effects of substance abuse and nonadherence to medication. *American Journal of Psychiatry*, 155 (2), 226–231, 1998.

Tarter, R., T. Blackson, J. Brigham, H. Moss, and G. Caprara, The association between childhood irritability and liability to substance use in early adolescence: A two year follow-up study of boys at risk for substance abuse. *Drug Alcohol Dependence*, 39, 253–261, 1995.

Thase, M.E., Long-term nature of depression. *Journal of Clinical Psychiatry*, 60 (supp. 14), 3–9, 1999.

Thase, M.E., C.F. Reynold III, E. Frank, A.D. Simons, G.D. Garamoni, J. McGeary, T. Harden, A.L. Fasiczka, and J.F. Cahalane, Response to cognitive behavior therapy in chronic depression. *Journal of Psychotherapy Practice and Research*, 3, 204–214, 1994.

Thase, M.E., and J.H. Wright, Cognitive-behavior therapy manual for depressed inpatients: A treatment protocol outline. *Behavior Therapy*, 22, 579–595, 1991.

Tomasson, K., and P. Vaglum, Psychiatric co-morbidity an aftercare among alcoholics: A prospective study of a nationwide representative sample. *Addiction*, 93 (3), 423–431, 1998.

Torrey, E.F., *Surviving Manic-Depressive Illness: A Guide to Bipolar Illness for Clients, Families, and Providers*. New York: Harper Collins, 2002.

Torrey, E.F., *Surviving Schizophrenia: A Manual for Families, Consumers, and Providers*, 4th ed. New York: Harper Collins, 2001.

U.S. Department of Health and Human Services, *Report to Congress on the Prevention and Treatment of Co-Occurring Substance Abuse Disorders and Mental Disorders*. Rockville, Maryland: USDHHS, 2002.

Valasquez, M.M., G.C. Maurer, C. Crouch, and C.C. DiClemente, *Group Treatment of Substance Abuse: A Stages-of-Change Therapy Manual*. New York: Guilford, 2001.

Verinis, J.S., and J. Taylor, Increasing alcoholic patients' aftercare attendance. *The International Journal of the Addictions*, 29 (11), 1487–1494, 1994.

Volkow, N.D., and J.S. Fowler, Addiction, a disease of compulsion and drive: involvement of the orbitofrontal cortex. *Cerebral Cortex*, 10, 318–325, 2000.

Walitzer, K.S., K.H. Dermen, and G.J. Connors, Strategies for preparing clients for treatment. *Behavior Modification*, 23 (1), 129–151, 1999.

Walker, R., D. Minor-Schork, R. Block, and J. Esinhart, High-risk factors for rehospitalization within six months. *Psychiatric Quarterly*, 67, 235–242, 1996.

Walsh, R., *Essential Spirituality*. New York: John Wiley, 1999.

Washton, A.M., ed., *Psychotherapy and Substance Abuse: A Practitioner's Handbook*. New York: Guilford, 1995.

Washton, A.M., Structured outpatient group treatment. In J.H. Lowinson, P. Ruiz, R.B. Millman, and J.G. Langrod, eds. *Substance Abuse: A Comprehensive Textbook*, 3rd ed. Baltimore, Maryland: Williams and Wilkins, 440–447, 1997.

Weiss, R.D., and D.C. Daley, *Understanding Personality Problems and Addiction*, 2nd ed. Center City, Minnesota: Hazelden, 2003.

Weiss, R.D., M.L. Griffin, S.F. Greenfield, L.M. Najavits, D. Wyner, J.A. Soto, and J.A. Hennen, Group therapy for patients with bipolar disorder and substance dependence: Results of a pilot study. *Journal of Clinical Psychiatry*, 61 (5), 361–367, 2000.

Weissman, M.M., J.C. Markowitz, and G.L. Klerman, *Comprehensive Guide to Interpersonal Psychotherapy*. New York: Basic Books, 2000.

Westermeyer, J.J., R.D. Weiss, and D.M. Ziedonis, eds., *Integrated Treatment for Mood and Substance Use Disorders*. Baltimore, Maryland: Johns Hopkins Press, 2003.

White, B.F., and J.A. MacDougall, *Clinician's Guide to Spirituality*. New York: McGraw-Hill Medical Publishing Division, 2001.

Wolpe, P.R., G. Gorton, R. Serota, and B. Sanford, Predicting compliance of dual diagnosis inpatients with aftercare treatment. *Hospital and Community Psychiatry*, 44 (1), 45–49, 1993.

Woody, G.E., Sociopathy and psychotherapy outcome. *Archives of General Psychiatry*, 42, 1081–1086, 1985.

Yalom, I.D., *The Theory and Practice of Group Psychotherapy*, 3rd ed. New York: Basic Books, 1985.

Ziedonis, D.M., and K. Trudeau, Motivation to quit using substances among individuals with schizophrenia: Implications for a motivation-based treatment. *Schizophrenia Bulletin*, 23 (2), 229–238, 1997.

Zuckoff, A., and D.C. Daley, Engagement and adherence issues in treating persons with non-psychosis dual disorders. *Psychiatric Rehabilitation Skills*, 5 (1), 131–162, 2001.

Zweben, A., and A. Zuckoff, Motivational interviewing and treatment adherence. In: W.R. Miller and S. Rollnick, eds. *Motivational Interviewing: Preparing People to Change Addictive Behavior,* 2nd ed. New York: Guilford, 2003.

Videos for Client and Family Education

Following is a list of videos available from Hazelden, Center City, Minnesota, *www.hazelden.com*; Gerald T. Rogers Productions, Wilmette, Illinois 1-800-227-9100; or *www.drdenniscdaley.com*. These videos focus on issues pertinent to recovery from substance use, psychiatric, or dual disorders. Most have written materials, such as workbooks, to help clients personalize the information presented. Videos can easily be incorporated in psychoeducational group sessions.

Wilmette, Illinois: Gerald T. Rogers Productions; Phone: 1-800-227-9100; *Living Sober Series*:

Balanced Living, 1997
Building a Recovery Network and Sponsorship, 1994
Compliance with Aftercare and Outpatient Counseling, 1999.
Compliance with Lifestyle Changes, 1999
Compliance with Medications and Self-Help Programs, 1999
Coping with Cravings and Thoughts of Using, 1994
Coping with Family and Interpersonal Conflict, 1994
Coping with Relapse Warning Signs, 1994
Double Trouble: Recovery from Chemical Dependency and Mental Illness,
    Part I—Mood and Anxiety, 1990
Double Trouble: Recovery from Chemical Dependency and Mental Illness,
    Part II—Personality Disorders, 1990
How to Sabotage Your Treatment
Low Motivation to Change or Seek Treatment, 1999
Managing Anger in Recover, 1994
Managing Feelings of Boredom and Emptiness, 1994
Motivation and Recovery, 1997
Other Addictions, 1997
Recovering from Crack/Cocaine Addiction, 1994
Relationship Issues: Part 1—Amends, Assertiveness, and Honest, 1997
Relationship Issues: Part 2—Passion, Rejection, and Criticism, 1997
Relationship Issues: Part 3—IIIV, Quick Sex, and Early Recovery Romances, 1997
Relationship to Therapist and Treatment Group, 1999
Resisting Social Pressures to Use Chemicals, 1992
Staying Sober, Keeping Straight, 1988
Together: Families in Recovery, 1989
Why Are You So Angry? 1991

Center City, Minnesota: Hazelden; *www.hazelden.org*
Preventing Relapse, 1994
Reflections from the Heart of a Child
Understanding Anxiety Disorders and Addiction, 1994
Understanding Bipolar Disorder and Addiction, 2003
Understanding Depression and Addiction. Center City, 1994

Understanding Personality Problems and Addiction, 2003
Understanding Schizophrenia and Addiction, 2003
Understanding Suicide and Addiction, 2003

Dr. Dennis C. Daley; *www.drdenniscdaley.com*
Developing A Relapse Plan, 1995
How to Use Therapy or Counseling, 1995
Psychiatric Illness and the Family, 1995
Recovering from Anxiety and Panic, 1995
Recovering from Bipolar Illness, 1995
Recovering from Borderline Personality Disorder, 1995
Recovering from Bulimia, 1995
Recovering from Depression, 1995
Recovering from Schizophrenia, 1995
The Role of Medication in Recovery, 1995
Understanding Psychiatric Illness and the Process of Recovery, 1995

World Wide Web-Based Resources

For more information on substance use, psychiatric, or dual disorders, you can go to the World Wide Web and search for a specific illness or topic. Following is a brief listing of Web resources.

Alcoholics Anonymous	www.alcoholic-anonymous.org
American Association of Suicidology	www.suicidology.org
American Psychiatric Association	www.psych.org
American Psychological Association	www.apa.org
Bipolar Disorders Portal	www.pendulum.org
CENAPS® (Terence T. Gorski)	www.cenaps.com
Depression and Related Affective Disorders Assoc.	www.med.jhu.edu
Dr. Dennis C. Daley	www.drdenniscdaley.com
Dr. Kenneth Minkoff	www.kenminkoff.com
Dual Recovery Anonymous (DRA)	www.dualrecovery.org
Dual Diagnosis Foundation	www.dualdiagnosis.org
Hazelden Educational Materials	www.hazelden.org
Mental Health Infosource	www.mhsource.com
Moodswing	www.moodswing.org
Narcotics Anonymous	www.na.org
National Alliance for the Mentally Ill	www.nami.org
National Clearinghouse for Alcohol and Drug Info.	www.ncadi.nih.gov
National Depressive and Manic-Depressive Assoc.	www.ndma.org
National Foundation for Depressive Illness, Inc.	www.depression.org
National Mental Health Association	www.nmha.org
Suicide Prevention Advocacy Network	www.spanusa.org
Support Group.Com Home Page	www.support-group.com